Keto Fat Loss
31 Ideas for Successfully Burning Fat

This book includes:

1) The Ketogenic Diet: *The Fast Way to Burning Fat*

*** 31 Ideas for Successfully Burning Fat**

Bonus Book

Intermittent Fasting: *The Smart Way to Losing Weight*

By Epic Rios

Intro

Thanks for purchasing *Keto Fat Loss: 31 Ideas for Successfully Burning Fat.*

In this book you will not only learn about the Ketogenic Diet but you will also learn 31 unique ideas for helping you with your fat loss goals.

I would highly recommend reading this book a few times especially the part that includes the 31 unique ideas for burning fat.

Learning about the Ketogenic Diet and how it can help you to live a healthier life is great.

But I truly believe the 31 unique ideas will give you a "bigger picture" of what is truly required to live healthy lifestyle.

In addition, making small positive changes every day will most certainly help you achieve your health and fitness goals.

One thing to keep in mind is that it is not enough to achieve your health and fitness goals. Instead, you want to make a commitment to live a better and healthier life every day of your life.

After you read this book a few times, make sure you apply what you have learned. In addition, use the 31 unique ideas as a guide to help you along your health and fitness journey.

One last thing, included with this book is *Intermittent Fasting: The Smart Way to Losing Weight.*

I have included this book as a way to thank you for purchasing my book.

Thanks again for purchasing *Keto Fat Loss: 31 Ideas for Successfully Burning Fat.*

I wish you great success with achieving your health and fitness goals.

The Ketogenic Diet

The Fast Way to Burning Fat

By Epic Rios

"Pursue your health and fitness goals diligently, patiently and persistently and you are bound to be successful." — *Epic Rios*

Table of Contents

© Copyright 2018 by __**Epic Rios**__ All rights reserved.

The following book is reproduced below with the goal of providing information that is as accurate and reliable as possible.

Regardless, purchasing this book can be seen as consent to the fact that both the publisher and the author of this book are in no way experts on the topics discussed within and that any recommendations or suggestions that are made herein are for entertainment purposes only.

Professionals should be consulted as needed prior to undertaking any of the action endorsed herein.

This declaration is deemed fair and valid by both the American Bar Association and the Committee of Publishers Association and is legally binding throughout the United States.

Furthermore, the transmission, duplication or reproduction of any of the following work including specific information will be considered an illegal act irrespective of if it is done electronically or in print.

This extends to creating a secondary or tertiary copy of the work or a recorded copy and is only allowed with express written consent from the Publisher. All additional right reserved.

The information in the following pages is broadly considered to be a truthful and accurate account of facts and as such any inattention, use or misuse of the information in question by the reader will render any resulting actions solely under their purview.

There are no scenarios in which the publisher or the original author of this work can be in any fashion deemed liable for any hardship or damages that may befall them after undertaking information described herein.

Additionally, the information in the following pages is intended only for informational purposes and should thus be thought of as universal. As befitting its nature, it is presented without assurance regarding its prolonged validity or interim quality.

Trademarks that are mentioned are done without written consent and can in no way be considered an endorsement from the trademark holder.

Introduction

Congratulations on purchasing this book and thank you for doing so. The following chapters will discuss what you need to know to get started on the ketogenic diet.

This diet plan is one of the best diet plans out there because it is effective and it helps you to lose weight and burn off that stubborn fat that you have been working against for a long time.

Simply this effective book will provide you with all of the information that you need to fully understand and follow the ketogenic diet plan.

We will start out with some of the basics of the ketogenic diet, the benefits of this diet plan, how to eat properly, the best meal plans to help you get started, how the ketogenic diet and intermittent fasting can work together, and even how you can modify this diet plan for your workout plan.

Anyone is able to follow the ketogenic diet, and with the help of this educational book, you will be able to see amazing results with your fat and weight loss in no time.

When you have been trying other diet plans for some time and are not seeing the results that you would like, it may be time to change things up and try something new.

The ketogenic diet will effectively help you to see the results that you would like, and this resourceful book will give you all the information that you need to get started.

I want to take the time to thank you so much for choosing this book! Every effort was made to ensure it is full of as much useful information as possible, please enjoy!

Chapter 1: What is the Ketogenic Diet?

When you are ready to get started on a new diet plan, there are a lot of different options that you can choose from.

Some diets are going to be more like "fasting" where you need to cut out what you eat so much that it is very hard to stick with it.

Other diets will focus on cutting out all of the fats that you consume during the day so that you can focus on eating healthy carbs and lots of fruits and vegetables in your diet.

Some diets are healthy and some are not that healthy and there are often many people who swear by these healthy and unhealthy diets.

But think about this, which diet is actually going to give you the best results that you would like to practice when it comes to losing weight?

It is important to state that the ketogenic diet is one of the most effective diet plans that you can choose from.

The ketogenic diet plan is simple to understand.

In addition, learning and practicing the ketogenic diet is going to take away some of the common misconceptions about dieting, the misconceptions that have been holding you back from losing weight so that you can actually achieve your fat loss goals.

While many traditional diets, the ones that are considered really healthy, will ask you to eat more carbs and cut down on fats, the ketogenic diet takes things in a different direction.

With the ketogenic diet, you are going to severely limit the carbs that you take in and instead replace them with healthy fats that will increase your metabolism and make you feel amazing in no time.

The issue with normal diet plans is that you are taking in too many carbs. These carbs may seem healthy, but when the body breaks them down, they basically become sugars in the body.

If you are consuming additional foods that have sugars in them then this could add some additional issues to your health and prevent you from achieving your weight loss goals.

Keep this in mind - the body is used to consuming carbs for energy. So, the body is very happy when you take in some carbs and the body will use the carbs for energy.

The body will then transfer the carbs over to insulin and then try to use up the insulin. And when the body doesn't use up all of its insulin, then the body simply stores it as fat. As a result, a person will simply gain weight or not be able to lose fat as a result of the excess insulin.

Unfortunately, carbs are a very effective source of energy for most people. The body will often feel hungry and run down long before you use up the carbs that you consume, and you will eventually feel tired, grumpy, and hungry again.

This leads most people to eat more carbs in an effort to get their energy back.

After eating more carbs, people will feel better for a little while. But soon they will be tired and worn out again and the cycle just keeps going on and on.

Eventually you will end up eating way too many calories just to keep your energy levels up and all those extra carbs will be stored as excess body fat.

The ketogenic diet works to break this cycle. Instead of relying so much on eating carbs, you will instead rely on eating healthy fats.

You can still have some carbs, but the point is to push your body into **ketosis, a process where the body will use fats instead of carbs as its main source of energy**.

It is important to state that fat or "healthy fat" can be a really efficient source of energy.

While you will feel worn out and tired for the first few days as the body runs out of carbs (due to you eating fewer carbs), and starts looking for a new energy source, you will soon notice that your energy levels will start to go through the roof.

You will burn the "healthy fat" that you are eating as well as the "fats" that are stored in the body, all while feeling full and satisfied.

When you go on the ketogenic diet, you are responsible for cutting down the number of carbs that you consume.

On the ketogenic diet, most people will be limited to eating no more than fifty grams of carbs each day. In addition, most of these carbs will come from healthy sources like fruits and vegetables.

Some people like to push themselves into ketosis a little bit faster and will limit themselves to twenty grams of carbs a day or less.

However, it is advisable to slowly begin the ketogenic diet and to also slowly begin to reduce the number of carbs you eat each day.

Every person that practices the ketogenic diet needs to experiment with their carb intake based on their activity levels and other factors.

For example, people who do a lot of weightlifting, aerobics and cardio based exercises (swimming, running, etc.,) will need to take in slightly more carbs or above the fifty-gram recommendation to help them stay healthy and so that they can maintain being in ketosis.

(Ketosis is a process by which the body uses stored fat or body fat as fuel or energy. So, when very little carbs are consumed and that energy is used up, the body will go into ketosis in which the body will look to fat as an energy source for using as fuel or energy.)

Checking to see if you are in ketosis is very important if you are practicing the ketogenic diet.

You will only lose weight once you reach the state of ketosis and some people may need to adjust their food intake a bit more than others to see some weight loss results.

It is important to state that there are test strips available at pharmacies that you can buy that will allow you to check for the level of ketones in your body, so that you can adjust your diet early on and figure out what changes you need to make to your diet.

(Ketones are chemical substances that the body produces when there is not enough insulin produced in the body as a result of eating very few carbs.

So, the less carbs you eat the less insulin your body will produce resulting in ketones being produced by the body. So, ketones occur as a result of the body using fat as energy or fuel.)

Remember that when working with the ketogenic diet, you need to change up the way that you are eating on a regular basis.

You are not going to be able to eat a ton of bread and pasta and see results. However, lots of healthy oils and fats from healthy protein sources can help you to get the macronutrients that you need and to lose weight.

Carbs are not completely off limits, but you will be surprised at how quickly your daily allowance will disappear, especially if you are choosing bread and pasta as your carb sources.

Instead, you need to stick with healthy fruits and vegetables and learn how to go with the ones that are lower in carb content compared to others.

This makes it easier to get the vitamins and nutrients that your body needs without pushing the body out of ketosis.

Once you reach ketosis through healthy fats, moderate amounts of protein, and low carbs, you will need to maintain this diet for the long-term. As soon as you start to eat more carbs and go back to your old habits, you will get out of ketosis and can start to gain the weight again.

You can easily lose a lot of weight with the ketogenic diet, but you need to maintain the ketosis diet for the long-term if you really want to see the good results.

Following the ketogenic diet can be a bit difficult for some people. You may have to give up some of the foods that you have enjoyed in the past.

But once you learn a few of the rules that come with the ketogenic diet and you find a few favorite recipes that will help you to stay within the right macronutrient content for your body and for ketosis you are going to fall in love with the results.

The ketogenic diet may be hard in our modern world, but it is going to give you some amazing results with your weight and fat loss goals.

Understanding Ketosis

Ketosis is basically the process of your body relying on fats rather than on carbs or glucose to provide it with energy.

Most people eat enough carbs that they are going to rely on those for their source of energy. But this is not a very efficient form of energy.

You will quickly go through cycles of high energy and then crash when the carbs are all gone, and you will end up eating way more than you need just to keep your energy levels up.

With ketosis, you do not need to worry about your energy levels crashing and then trying to eat more carbs in order to increase your energy levels again.

Instead, you will teach the body to stop relying on carbs and instead the body will learn to rely on healthy fats that you start to take in.

When you eat healthy fats, ketones are going to be produced and used for energy.

Ketones will replace the glucose, giving you plenty of healthy energy without having to worry about the horrible crashes that glucose (sugars from carbs) causes.

Eating on the Ketogenic Diet

When you follow a ketogenic diet, you will consume at least 70 percent of your calories each day from fat.

The majority of the rest will come from protein, with only about five percent coming from healthy sources of carbs, such as low-carb vegetables.

As a beginner, you will need to build your meals around healthy sources of fats. These can include oils, cheese, nuts, meats, and fatty fish.

You can then add in some healthy sources of protein if they are not included already, as well as healthy low-carb options like vegetables and some fruits.

One thing to keep in mind on this diet plan is that you still need to take in moderate amounts of protein.

Many people get so focused on the fat intake and limiting their carbs that they forget to take in enough protein.

Protein is important to help you stay full and for preserving your body's muscles as well as keeping your muscles strong.

Negative Effects of This Diet Plan

You may also wonder if there are any negative effects of following this diet plan. Plain and simple, you are taking a large food group (carbs) and cutting it down to almost nothing on this diet plan.

For the most part, as soon as your body has time to adapt to ketosis, there shouldn't be any negative effects that you need to deal with.

You may feel a bit tired in the beginning as your body adapts, but once that adaption happens, you will find that you have more energy than ever before.

You should make sure that you have a wide variety of food options when it comes to eating on the ketogenic diet plan.

If you eat the same meals each day, or the same vegetables, you are going to miss out on important nutrients and this can cause some negative effects.

This is true of any diet plan if you do not add in variety. Make sure that you get plenty of variety in the diet, and you will see amazing results without any negative side effects.

Do I Need to Measure Ketones?

Many people choose to monitor the ketones that they consume. Actually, it is important that you monitor your ketones in order to ensure that you reach ketosis and that you stay within it to see weight loss results.

It is not necessarily a requirement for the diet plan, but it certainly helps. Measuring your ketones does not have to be difficult.

There are some testing strips that you can use that will tell you when you have entered ketosis and you can bring these out any time that you are worried about whether you are in the right range with your carbs or not.

Who Uses the Ketogenic Diet?

The biggest reason that people will choose to go on the ketogenic diet is to simply lose weight.

When you start relying on fat for your source of energy rather than glucose (sugars), you can melt off the weight and fat in no time.

However, there are many other reasons that people may choose to practice the ketogenic diet.

Originally, the ketogenic diet was designed to help patients who were dealing with a variety of neurological conditions, especially epilepsy.

It was found that young children who relied on a ketogenic-like diet were able to reduce the frequency of their seizures and reduce their medications.

Believe it or not, but there are some athletes who like to use the ketogenic diet to help with their endurance.

According to a paper that was released in the European Journal of Clinical Nutrition, there are a few other reasons that someone may choose to use the ketogenic diet.

These include:

- Evidence that the ketogenic diet can help people with high cholesterol, type 2 diabetes, weight loss, and epilepsy.

- New evidence has shown how the ketogenic diet may be able to help with a variety of neurological diseases like brain trauma, narcolepsy, Alzheimer's, and Parkinson's Disease, to name a few.

- People that suffer from cancer, severe acne, and even polycystic ovarian syndrome are often helped with the ketogenic diet as well.

Basically, anyone is able to use the ketogenic diet, whether they want to lose weight or are working to avoid one of the conditions named above.

The ketogenic diet is easy to follow and gives such amazing benefits to those who are able to follow it.

Chapter 2: The Benefits of the Ketogenic Diet

There are a lot of reasons that people will choose to use and practice the ketogenic diet. Simply, the ketogenic diet is one of the most effective diet plans out there.

In addition, the ketogenic diet can help resolve a variety of health issues that people are dealing with and not just with weight loss.

Some of the great benefits that you will receive when you decide to use and practice the ketogenic diet are:

- **Lose weight:** The number one reason that people choose to use the ketogenic diet is that they want to lose weight. And this diet plan is very effective at helping this to happen.

  Once your body enters into the process of ketosis and starts relying on fats for energy rather than carbs, you will see the weight melt off in no time.

- **Next, the ketogenic diet can help reduce cancer:** Some studies have shown how the ketogenic diet may be effective at reducing your risks of developing cancer.

  Cancer cells thrive when given lots of carbs, so if you take these carbs away, they will basically starve out. Regular healthy cells can rely on healthy fats for their nutrition, but cancer cells can't.

- **Next, the ketogenic diet will give you more energy:** During the first few days on the ketogenic diet, you may notice that you are feeling tired and worn down. This is because the body is so used to relying on carbs to stay energetic.

  When you take those carbs away, the body is not sure where to find its energy source and may feel run down.

You just need to give it a few days, though; the body will start using the fats that you provide it for energy in no time. Once that happens, you will have more energy than ever before.

- **Next, the ketogenic diet will help lower your risk of diabetes:** With all those carbs you traditionally eat, it is common to see a risk of diabetes.

  You have to be very careful of the carbs you eat because the body will treat some carbs you eat just like sugars once they are eaten and broken down.

  So, if you are eating some sugars and lots of carbs, you are raising your insulin levels and increasing the amount of risk you have for diabetes.

  Cut out a lot of those carbs, as well as the sugars, and your body can clean itself up and cut down on your risk of diabetes.

- **Next, the ketogenic diet will lower your blood pressure:** Many people who have gone on the ketogenic diet report that their blood pressures went down.

  Many of the foods that you consume on a regular diet will have a ton of sodium inside, which can raise your blood pressure.

  Add in all the processed foods, high amount of carbs, and even the bad fats, and it is no wonder that most people have bad high blood pressure.

  The ketogenic diet cuts out a lot of these bad unhealthy foods out of your diet so that you can recover and get that blood pressure back to normal.

- **Next, the ketogenic diet is great for the heart:** The ketogenic diet can even help out with the health of your heart.

  The healthy fats that you consume will help to strengthen your heart. The healthy fats also deliver some of those healthy vitamins and nutrients over to the heart better than carbs do.

  So, once you are reducing some of the carbs, the ones that turn into sugars in the body, you are giving the heart a fighting chance to be healthy and strong again.

- **Next, the ketogenic diet clears the mind:** When you are able to cut down on the number of carbs that you consume, and the number of calories that you are consuming, you will find that your mind feels much clearer.

  It will feel amazing to remember things, to think things through critically, and to no longer have to deal with the brain fog that you may have suffered from before as a result of eating so many carbs.

- **Next, the ketogenic diet can help fight epilepsy:** Originally, the ketogenic diet was developed as a way to help children who were suffering from chronic epilepsy.

  The high fat and low carb ketogenic diet were effective at helping young children fight off epilepsy and kept the episodes away.

  The ketogenic diet needed to be used over the long-term, usually for two years or more, but helped children to not have to deal with the horrible effects of their seizures and helped them to reduce the amount of medication they needed to take.

Almost everyone is able to benefit from the use of the ketogenic diet.

It is different compared to some of the other diet plans that are available on the market, but this is part of what makes it so successful compared to the other diet plans.

When you are ready to start losing weight and improving many other aspects of your health, then make sure to try out the ketogenic diet to help you out.

Chapter 3: The Side Effects of the Ketogenic Diet

Before you get started with the ketogenic diet, it is important to know that there are some side effects or using and practicing the ketogenic diet.

These side effects are not horrible side effects like what you may be used to with common medications, but it is still a good idea to know what to expect when you are getting started on this new diet plan.

Some of the side effects that you may encounter when you are on the ketogenic diet are:

Dizziness or Headaches

One of the first side effects that you may experience when you get started with the ketogenic diet includes dizziness and headaches.

Dizziness and headaches are really prevalent in those individuals who for a very long time consumed a lot of caffeine and sugar before starting the ketogenic diet.

Both caffeine and sugar are highly addictive and if you go cold turkey on them, you may have a few side effects during the beginning process of the ketogenic diet.

You may introduce a little caffeine or sugar later on in the ketogenic diet plan if you want, but for those individuals who experience having a lot of trouble starting this diet plan or who really are addicted to caffeine and sugar, it is best to cut them out completely.

The good news is that the symptoms of withdrawal are only going to last for a few days and they really are not that severe.

You may feel a little anxious or upset because you will crave the caffeine and sugars that you are trying to eliminate from your diet.

However, if you are able to overcome your cravings for caffeine and sugar during the initial process of the ketogenic diet, you will break the addictions and you will not feel so reliant on consuming them as much.

One thing that you may decide to try is to slowly cut out your sugar and caffeine intake before you go on the ketogenic diet.

This will help you to not have to deal with these withdrawal symptoms as much. This can make things easier since you will already be dealing with feeling tired as your body gets used to the fats instead of the carbs.

If you are thinking about going on the ketogenic diet, consider cutting down on the sugars and caffeine for at least a few weeks ahead of time and you will not have to deal with the headaches or the dizziness as much when you begin.

Leg Cramps

Some of those who decide to go on the ketogenic diet will complain of dealing with leg cramps, especially when they are trying to go to bed at night.

This is common when you are in the early phase of the ketogenic diet.

This is a big problem for those users who are not paying attention to their micronutrients on this diet plan and who are not taking in enough potassium on this diet plan.

There are a few things that you are able to do to make sure you are getting enough potassium.

You can first work to try and eat plenty of foods with healthy amounts of potassium in them.

If you are having trouble doing this, you may decide to take a supplement that has potassium inside of it.

Many beginners decide to take a potassium supplement to help prevent leg cramps because keeping track of the macronutrients and the micronutrients for good health can be difficult.

However, you need to work towards not depending on supplements and instead eat real foods that will provide you with all the nutrients your body needs without taking any supplements.

Constipation

If you are not watching your micronutrients when you are on the ketogenic diet, you may deal with the issue of constipation.

This can be really uncomfortable for most people to deal with and can make sticking with the ketogenic diet a bit difficult.

However, the solution to this problem is pretty simple.

To ensure that you are not going to deal with constipation on the ketogenic diet plan, make sure that the majority of carbs that you decide to eat come from healthy green vegetables, which are full of fiber.

You also need to drink a lot of water on this diet plan because water has been shown to combat and prevent constipation.

For those individuals who maybe are already dealing with constipation, you may try a laxative to help you out.

Bad Breath

Another side effect that you may need to deal with on the ketogenic diet is bad breath.

While on the ketogenic diet plan, the body is going to burn up fat so that you can use this fat as energy.

This is the process of ketosis and will help you to burn through fat in your diet and the fat that is sitting around your body.

Unfortunately, the ketones (burning fat used as energy) that are released in this process will leave you with bad breath and make your urine smell bad.

The smell is going to be a little bit different than you may experience when after eating smelly food or by those individuals who suffer from halitosis (bad breath resulting from health problems).

Some people even compare it to a fruity candy smell instead, but if you do not want your breath to smell at all, then it is important to find a few ways to get rid of the bad breath.

Chewing on some gum without sugar, using mouthwash, or chewing on parsley or mint can help to get rid of this smell while keeping you on the ketogenic diet.

Feeling Tired

There are many people who will get started on the ketogenic diet who claim they feel tired.

They get going on this plan and are excited about all the big promises of more energy when they eat more healthy fats and fewer carbs.

Then they start on this diet and the first few days or in the first week they will begin to feel really tired almost like they just don't have enough energy to get things done.

This is completely normal on the ketogenic diet and it is important to know that these energy lacking feelings are going to fade away pretty soon.

The reason that you feel so tired when you start the ketogenic diet is that the body basically doesn't have any fuel for energy.

Sure, you are taking in healthy foods and providing it with fuel, but the body is used to relying on carbs and doesn't know what it should do when you take the majority of those carbs away.

So, the body is basically searching around hoping that you will eat and take in the carbs that it needs for easy energy access.

When you don't eat carbs or consume enough carbs your body is basically working on very little to no energy for a little while.

The good news is that feeling tired is not going to last for a very long time. For most people, it takes less than a week for the body to start recognizing the fat as a good source of energy and it will switch over.

Once the body starts to realize that it can use fat for energy instead of carbs, you will start to notice a big change.

Your energy will come back in a big way and you will feel amazing in no time.

You will be able to keep going all day long, even with fewer calories, and will ensure that you feel great about this diet plan.

As you can see, none of these side effects are life-threatening or that big of a deal when it comes to the ketogenic diet.

These side effects can make you a little bit uncomfortable and may not be the most pleasant when you are dealing with bad breath and feeling tired.

However, these side effects will usually not last for a long time and once your body adjusts to the ketogenic diet plan, you will not have to worry about them any longer.

Chapter 4: Who Can Safely Go on the Ketogenic Diet?

In most cases, following the ketogenic diet is a great experience. There are so many great health benefits that you will be able to enjoy when it comes to the ketogenic diet.

Many people choose to go on the ketogenic diet because they are tired of not being able to lose weight or fight off all that excess fat that has been hanging around their body for a long time.

But weight loss is not the only reason that you may choose to go on the ketogenic diet. If you have been fighting diabetes and its side effects for some time, reducing the number of carbs and the glucose it produces can help combat this health issue.

If you are worried about your high cholesterol levels and high blood pressure, simply practicing and following the ketogenic diet plan can help you to reduce your risks with these health issues as well.

Even younger children who have been dealing with epilepsy and those children with other neurological conditions may be able to benefit with the help of the ketogenic diet.

The children may be able to reduce some of the symptoms that they are dealing with and some have even been able to no longer need to use the medication they are on when they accurately follow the ketogenic diet plan.

Anyone who is dealing with health diseases or wants to lose weight or just simply wants to live a healthier lifestyle will be able to discover that the ketogenic diet is a good tool to help them out.

It doesn't matter if you are a man or a woman, the ketogenic diet is the right option to help anyone.

Who Shouldn't Use the Ketogenic Diet?

There are so many people who are able to use the ketogenic diet. The ketogenic diet has a lot of benefits and it can help you to lose weight, fight off many health concerns, and help you to feel amazing in no time.

However, there are certain groups of people who should avoid and not practice the ketogenic diet.

Practicing the ketogenic diet plan can be detrimental to the health of some people and even make them feel sick.

Some of those individuals who should avoid the ketogenic diet are:

- Children and teenagers
- Women who are pregnant and breastfeeding
- Women with irregular menstrual cycles
- People that have issues with their thyroid glands
- People that suffer from adrenal fatigue
- High-level athletes who need carbs to help them function better

These groups of people will often not do as well with the ketogenic diet.

This is because they need special dietary requirements that are eliminated from their diet when they follow the ketogenic diet.

For example, a pregnant or nursing mother needs to take in carbs to help her baby to grow and eliminating these completely can result in a nutrient deficiency for the baby.

Teenagers and children often need some of the glucose that is found in carbs, or they need higher carb content from fruits and vegetables than the ketogenic diet allows.

This does not mean that these groups of people can't take some advice from the ketogenic diet to help them stay healthy.

For example, teenagers or pregnant women may choose to limit their carbs a bit, but not to the fifty grams a day that is recommended by the ketogenic diet.

Instead, teenagers or pregnant women can instead stick to eating healthy carbs like fruits and vegetables while reducing their intake of unhealthy carbs like the bread and pastas that they normally eat.

Teenagers or pregnant women can also consider increasing their healthy fat intake and eating good amounts of protein each day.

So basically, some of these groups of people can follow some of the principles of the ketogenic diet without following or practicing so many of the restrictions the actual diet requires.

If you fall into one of the groups above, it may be a good idea to talk to your doctor before attempting to go on this diet plan.

This will help you to determine if you really need the ketogenic diet and if it is actually a healthy option for you, especially if you are in one of the groups above.

Chapter 5: The Ketogenic Diet and Exercise

It is important to understand how exercise and your fitness performance can be affected by the ketogenic diet.

It is also important to understand that maybe your exercise routine/plan/goals may need to be changed a little bit as a result of practicing the ketogenic diet.

However, you will still see some great results from your fitness workouts while practicing the ketogenic diet.

In additional, habitual exercise combined with the ketogenic diet will help you to lose weight and fat faster than ever.

You may also need to add a few extra carbs to your diet in order to have the right amount of energy for achieving your health and fitness goals.

With the ketogenic diet, you are greatly reducing the number of carbs that you are consuming and since many athletes require carbs to help them stay energetic, you may be curious to know how this is going to affect your body when you enter ketosis.

You will need to keep a few things in mind when you get started on the ketogenic diet when it comes to exercising, but it is just fine to exercise on this diet and all the health benefits definitely make it worth your time.

First, we need to understand that the traditional view on weight loss, the idea that you just need to eat less and exercise for a longer period of time (while getting plenty of cardio in as well) is advice that is outdated and just won't work with the ketogenic diet.

To really lose weight and get that leaner frame that you have been looking for, the foods that you eat while on the ketogenic diet are what matter the most.

Eating recommended foods on the ketogenic diet like meats, seafood, and dairy are great ways to begin the ketogenic diet.

The most important thing you can do for weight loss and maintaining your energy levels is to pay attention to how well and how disciplined you are to following the ketogenic diet.

If you are able to remain in a steady state of ketosis, rather than coming in and out of it because you can't keep your carbs steady or low, you will see some amazing results.

Before you decide to start doing more and more of your regular physical exercise activities while on the ketogenic diet, make sure that you understand when your body is in ketosis as well as spend some time testing your ketone levels.

However, once you get used to how the ketogenic diet works, adding in exercise can provide you with a lot of good benefits to your health.

Physical exercise like strength training and lifting weights will help to make your bones stronger as well as build muscle and make you have that lean look you want.

In addition, physical exercise like strength training and lifting weights is also great for the heart.

And as long as you are taking in nutrients properly on the ketogenic diet, physical exercise can easily fit in with your new diet plan.

Just remember that when you are exercising while on the ketogenic diet, make sure to stay healthy, make sure your energy levels are good and don't harm yourself while practicing the ketogenic diet.

Why Should I Exercise on the Ketogenic Diet?

After learning a bit more about ketosis and how the body needs higher levels of carbs in order to properly perform the activities that you would like, you may think that ketosis is not the best for long-term exercise.

However, exercising while on the ketogenic diet actually provides the user with many benefits including:

- In one study, ultra-endurance athletes were asked to do a three-hour run.

  Those who ate a low carb diet for about twenty months on average had up to three times the fat burn compared to the athletes who followed a high-carb diet.

  Both of these groups were able to replenish the same amount of muscle glycogen when done.

- Studies have shown that ketosis can help to prevent fatigue in people who exercise for long periods of time.

  For example, people that strength train for 1 or 2 hours or people who do cardio exercise activities such as running have sufficient energy to complete their long workouts.

- Ketosis is great for helping to maintain your blood glucose levels, whether you are considered obese or not.

- With the help of keto-adaption (which we will talk about later on), low-carb ketogenic dieters are actually better able to perform various activities, even while taking in fewer carbs over time.

- You receive all the regular benefits of exercise. In addition to the benefits listed above, those individuals who are on the ketogenic diet are able to receive all the same benefits that they would receive on any other diet while working out.

  However, the main difference between the ketogenic diet and other diets is that the ketogenic diet uses fat as energy instead of carbs.

  Keep this in mind, exercising while on the ketogenic diet will help you to be in a better mood, lose weight, see fat loss, control your blood sugar levels, reduce blood pressure, and so much more.

  Everyone should consider starting on their own workout program and combining it with the ketogenic diet.

  It is important to state that having a good mixture of different exercises, from flexibility to strength training and some lower-intensity aerobics or cardio exercises, will help you to make the whole body strong and will prevent injuries along the way.

While you may need to take a little bit of time off from working out when you first get started with the ketogenic diet to help you adjust, most people are able to successfully work out while practicing the ketogenic diet.

By making a few adjustments to your ketogenic lifestyle and by watching how many carbs you eat as well as when you consume your carbs will make all the difference in the results that you see when it comes to achieving your weight loss goals.

Types of Exercises to do While on the Ketogenic Diet

Your nutritional needs are going to vary based on the exercise or exercises that you want to perform. But generally, you will be able to divide up exercises into four group.

These four groups of exercises include stability training, flexibility training, anaerobic exercises, and aerobic exercises.

Let's take a look at how each of these can work with the ketogenic diet:

- **Aerobic exercise:** Aerobic exercise is typically known as cardio (swimming, running, cycling) and it will be any activity that gets the heart up and running for more than three minutes.

  As a result, your body may require more carbs while practicing the ketogenic diet.

  If you do cardio exercises that are steady-state and lower in intensity like walking you are going to be concentrating on fat burning, which makes it a great exercise for the ketogenic diet.

- **Anaerobic exercise:** This type of exercise is going to have short bursts of energy throughout an exercise session, such as HIIT, powerlifting or explosive exercises.

  If you plan to do anaerobic exercises, you may need to take in more carbs because anaerobic exercises require a lot more carbs as their primary fuel source.

Make sure that when you combine anaerobic exercises with the ketogenic diet that you consume just a little more carbs just for the sake of making sure you have the necessary energy to complete your physical workouts.

- **Flexibility training:** It is a good idea to add some flexibility exercises to your fitness routine.

  Flexibility training can be helpful for stretching out the muscles, improving your range of motion, and supporting the joints.

  Flexibility training is often used to help prevent injuries from some of the other workouts that you may do.

  Some examples of flexibility training are Yoga and just simple stretching exercises.

  Flexibility training does not require a lot of carbs. As a result, the ketogenic diet is perfect for people that do Yoga or simple stretching exercises.

- **Stability exercises:** Stability exercises are exercises that work on your core or abdominal (abs) muscles as well as help improve your balance.

  Stability exercises are good for helping control your body's movements, strengthen the muscles in the body, and can even improve your body's alignment.

  Stability exercises do not require a lot of carbs.

  As a result, the ketogenic diet is perfect for people that practice stability exercises.

Keep this in mind when you are exercising while practicing the ketogenic diet:

"Mix up your workouts as much as possible. Do a combination of all four types of exercises and or training mentioned above for the purpose of developing the type of body that you want.

At the same time always monitor your energy levels to make sure you are consuming just enough carbs while practicing the ketogenic diet.

If at any moment you are feeling too tired to complete your workout routine simply stop exercising, monitor your energy levels and see if you need to increase your carbs intake. Safety first."

It is important to state that as you practice the ketogenic diet and you reach ketosis, the intensity of your exercise workouts is going to matter quite a bit.

When you do low-intensity workouts like walking or Yoga, the body will rely more on fat as its energy source, so these workouts are the best for those on the ketogenic diet.

The high-intensity aerobic exercises, like jogging and running, and anaerobic exercises, like powerlifting and sprinting, are going to rely more on carbs as an energy source and are not the best exercises to do while practicing the ketogenic diet.

Just keep in mind that if you are going to do high-intensity exercises you may need to add some more carbs to your diet.

Picking a Targeted Ketogenic Diet (Variations)

So far, we have just been talking about the basic ketogenic diet. This is a great diet if you are looking to get started and you don't plan to do really intense workouts.

The ketogenic diet will often work for regular exercise and for a little bit of low-intensity activities as well.

But if you are planning on doing activities that are more intense, or you plan to exercise or workout more than three days out of the week to help with weight and fat loss, then it is time to consider a targeted ketogenic diet variation.

A targeted ketogenic diet variation will help you to adjust your diet so that you get enough carbs to help you achieve your fitness goals as well as keep you in ketosis.

Those higher intensity workouts, like lots of weightlifting and sprinting are not going to do well with the regular ketogenic diet so having a targeted ketogenic diet variation will help you get the results that you would like.

These targeted ketogenic diet variations will allow you to have some more carbs during the day so that you can maintain your activity levels.

This does not mean that you can go out and enjoy as many sodas and baked goods as you like.

You still need to get your carbs from keto approved foods, like fruits and vegetables, but you are allowed to increase your healthy carb intake.

A good thing to remember is that you should eat about 15 to 30 grams of fast acting carbs (which includes options like fruit) about twenty minutes before and after your workout.

This helps your muscles to get the glycogen that they need to do well during training and so that your muscles can recover.

Eating during that time period will ensure that the carbs are used for the workout, so you won't leave ketosis at all.

Options or Variations of the Ketogenic Diet

There are a few options for the ketogenic diet that you can pick based on the amount of physical activity that you plan to do.

The different ketogenic diet variations that you can choose from include:

- **The standard ketogenic diet:** With this diet option you will keep your total carb count between 20 to 50 grams each day.

- **The targeted ketogenic diet:** With this diet option, you will stick with the 20 to 50 grams of carbs each day. But you will plan out when you eat these carbs.

  You will want to get the majority, if not all, of these carbs about an hour or less before you do your exercise. This is the best option for athletes who like to do high-intensity activities like weightlifting, sprinting, CrossFit, etc.,

- **The cyclical ketogenic diet:** For this one, you will cut your carbs down to almost nothing for a few days.

  And then on the days that you want to do a higher-intensity workout, you will eat higher-carbs on that day. This should even out for the right amount of carbs throughout the week.

Depending on the exercises that you are doing you may find that the carb content is too low, and you are not taking in enough carbs to keep up with your activity levels.

If you want to know if you are in a state of ketosis, you can simply purchase some test strips at the local pharmacy that will help you to know whether you are in ketosis or not.

You may also be able to increase your carb intake a little bit and still remain in the state of ketosis.

However, it is important to be careful when you slightly increase your carbs intake because it is really easy to jump out of ketosis.

In addition, if you do jump out of ketosis then you will lose the benefits of the ketogenic diet plan if you aren't closely monitoring how many carbs you consume.

The good news is that most people are able to adapt to eating lower-carb diets and using fat to help them get the fuel that they need.

This may take a few weeks and you may not be as strong for those first few weeks as the body adjusts. However, the longer you remain on the ketogenic diet, the more the body can adapt to this diet plan.

After practicing the ketogenic diet for a while, your body will become more efficient at burning the fat and using up the ketones that are in the body.

With enough physical exercise and after a while of being on the ketogenic diet, you will be able to see some amazing results with your body as well as achieve whatever fitness goals you plan to achieve.

Chapter 6: What Should I Eat on the Ketogenic Diet?

One question that a lot of people will ask when getting started on the ketogenic diet is what they are allowed to eat.

Working with the right macronutrients is one of the most important parts of the ketogenic diet. You must make sure that you are eating plenty of healthy fats and low carbs so that you can stay in ketosis.

Actually, eating plenty of healthy fats and low carbs is going to be one of the most important things that you concentrate on when it comes to the ketogenic diet.

However, as long as the foods that you eat fit into these macronutrients, and you are getting plenty of vitamins and minerals from the fruits and vegetables you choose to eat, you will lose weight.

Before we look at the specific foods that you are able to eat on the ketogenic diet let's take a look at the macronutrients.

This is really important and will ensure that you are eating enough fats to stay energetic as well as keeping the carbs low enough so that you don't kick yourself out of ketosis.

Also, don't forget that it is important to eat healthy sources of protein rich foods so that you can keep your muscles big and strong.

First, let's take a look at the fats that you need to eat. It is recommended that you get somewhere between 70 to 75 percent of your daily calories from healthy fats.

You must make sure that these are healthy fats. Going to the local fast food restaurant and eating a big burger and fries will not count because these are bad fats that will not help out with the ketogenic diet.

Instead, eating healthy fats like olive oil, fats from dairy products, and fats that come in healthy protein sources are much better options.

You will also need to eat moderate amounts of protein as well. You will need between 15 and 20 percent of your daily calories from protein.

This helps to keep the muscles as strong as possible and can be especially important if you are someone who likes to work out a lot and wants to build muscle with the ketogenic diet plan. Stick with options like healthy fish, chicken, turkey, and ground beef.

And finally, most people will want to keep their carb intake down to five percent or lower. If you are really into weight lifting, you can sometimes go up to ten percent.

But, before you increase your carbs intake, make sure that you experiment and see if you are really in ketosis with the higher amount of carbs or not.

Remember, when choosing carbs to eat stick with healthy options like fruits and vegetables that will help to keep you feeling full.

In addition, eating healthy carbs like fruits and vegetables will give your body the vitamins and nutrients that your body needs.

If you are able to stick with these macronutrients, you will see great results with the ketogenic diet.

It will take some time to get used to which foods will fit into this diet plan, but once you get used to it, losing weight and fat will be easier than ever before.

Foods to Eat on the Ketogenic Diet

Sticking with the macronutrients that we talked about above is one of the most important things that you can do on this diet plan.

But putting this into a meal plan can be difficult when you first get started.

Some of the foods that you are able to enjoy when following the ketogenic diet include:

- **Meat:** There are many different types of meat that you can enjoy, and this will provide you with the protein and some of the fats that you need.

You can choose from options like fish, lamb, veal, pork, venison, chicken, quail, duck, and shellfish.

With chicken, make sure that you leave the skin on to help increase the fat content, but do not bread or batter any poultry that you eat.

Make sure that you do not eat any processed meats, though. If choosing canned fish options, make sure that the preservation method does not use any added sugar.

- **Eggs:** Many meals on the ketogenic diet will require you to eat eggs for the purpose of consuming both protein and healthy fat.

  Because eggs have lots of healthy protein and fats, they can be eaten for breakfast, lunch or dinner.

- **Cheese:** For the most part, cheese is a good food to eat while on the ketogenic diet. There are a few carbs found in the different varieties of cheese, so make sure to read the labels carefully and then count the carbs before you eat them.

Some cheese may push you over your daily required carbs intake so make sure you keep track of other carbs you have eaten that day.

- **Vegetables:** Vegetables will contain most of the carbs that you are going to eat but try to keep this to a minimum.

  You should go with the green and leafy options because these are lower in carbs so options like lettuce, cabbage, kale, and watercress are great.

  You can also go with options like bean sprouts, cucumber, celery, broccoli, and asparagus.

- **Fruits:** You can enjoy some fruits on the ketogenic diet, but you need to be careful about which ones you eat.

  Some fruits can be higher in carbs compared to some of the other food options on the list and if you eat too many fruits, you will end up going over your daily required carbs intake.

  If you choose to add some fruits to your diet, carefully watch your portions and avoid going over on the carb content.

  One recommended fruit is the avocado. The avocado is a good source of healthy fat so try to make the avocado part of your ketogenic diet meal plan.

- **Nuts:** Nuts are a good source of healthy fats and protein so they are fine to eat as long as you eat them in moderation as a type of dessert or as a snack. Some recommended nuts are walnuts.

- **Cream, butter, and oils** are usually fine because they provide you with some healthy sources of fat.

- **Dry spices** and **fresh herbs** are great for the ketogenic diet. Dry spices and fresh herbs will help you to get some flavoring in your meals without adding in any extra carbs.

As you can see, while you do need to be careful with the macronutrients that you are consuming on the ketogenic diet, there are still some options that you can go with to eat great meals.

Mix and match some of the options that were mentioned above, and you will get tasty meals that are easy to make and will help you to lose weight without feeling hungry.

Foods to Avoid on the Ketogenic Diet

For the most part, if the foods are not listed in the section above, you should not consume them on the ketogenic diet.

Consuming foods that are not recommended for the ketogenic diet can add in too many bad fats, bad carbs, and sugars than your body does not need.

In addition, consuming foods that are not recommended for the ketogenic diet may kick you out of your ketosis state.

Keep in mind that you do not want to work hard to get into ketosis and then end up cheating yourself and getting kicked out of ketosis because you consumed foods that are not recommended for the ketogenic diet.

Some of the foods that you will need to avoid on the ketogenic diet are:

- **Bread and pasta:** Bread and pasta may seem healthy, but just a small serving can put you over your required daily carb intake.

There are healthier alternatives, such as keto bread or using vegetables to make noodles, so you can still enjoy some of your favorite meals without having to worry about eating too many carbs.

- **Baked goods:** In between the excess carbs and sugars that are inside most baked goods, it is no wonder that baked goods are not allowed on the ketogenic diet.

  It is best to stick with eating a piece of fruit (especially if you can find one that is lower in carbs) for your snack rather than eating any of the baked goods that are available.

- **Processed frozen foods/meals:** Anything that you can find in the freezer section of your grocery store should be avoided.

  These may seem healthy, but the preservatives and carbs are extremely high and will kick you out of ketosis.

  It is best to just leave everything that is in the freezer section alone and stick with fresh and whole foods instead.

- **Sodas:** Some people choose to drink diet sodas when they are on the ketogenic and diet sodas are allowed. However, you should avoid regular sodas because of all the sugar that is inside of them.

- **Fast foods:** While you are on the ketogenic diet, you need to avoid going out to eat.

  Fast foods are full of way too many carbs and bad fats and will instantly take you out of ketosis without much effort. Avoid fast foods and just cook your meals at home instead.

- **Deli meats:** Deli meats may seem like a good option to get your protein, but in reality, they are mostly processed and full of lots of carbs.

  It is best to avoid deli meats as much as possible and focus your time and energy on eating healthier proteins and carbs.

It is important that you eat the right foods when it comes to the ketogenic diet.

There are some other diet plans that will allow you to cheat on occasion, but when you cheat on the ketogenic diet, you lose all of your weight loss benefits.

If you would like to stay in ketosis and really lose weight, then make sure to avoid the foods mentioned above and you will see great results with the ketogenic diet.

Chapter 7: Simple Meal Plans for the Ketogenic Diet

One of the hardest things that many beginners have trouble with is figuring out what they need to eat on the ketogenic diet.

While they may understand how the macronutrients are supposed to work on the diet, they are worried about how to plan out their meals and how to make it work well for them.

Coming up with ideas for your ketogenic meal plans is one of the best things that you can do because it outlines what you need to eat for the whole week or longer if you like.

Now, we are going to look at a simple one-week meal plan that you can follow to get started on the ketogenic diet and see amazing results in no time.

Monday
Breakfast: Scrambled Eggs
Lunch: Keto Asian Salad
Dinner: Pesto Chicken Casserole

Tuesday
Breakfast: Cheese Roll-ups
Lunch: Egg Omelet
Dinner: Meat Pie

Wednesday
Breakfast: Frittata with Spinach
Lunch: Chicken Soup (No Noodle)
Dinner: Carbonara

Thursday
Breakfast: Dairy Free Latte
Lunch: Avocado and Goat Cheese Salad
Dinner: Keto Pizza

Friday
Breakfast: Mushroom Omelet
Lunch: Smoked Salmon
Dinner: Keto Tacos

Saturday
Breakfast: Baked Bacon Omelet
Lunch: Keto Quesadillas
Dinner: Asian Stir-Fry

Sunday
Breakfast: Berry Pancakes
Lunch: Italian Keto Plate
Dinner: Pork Chops

Keto Recipes

Recipe #1
Scrambled Eggs with Spinach
What's in it?
- Some salt
- Pepper
- Butter (1 oz.)
- Eggs (2)
- Spinach

How's it done?
Whisk together the eggs while adding the pepper and salt.

Add some butter to a skillet and let it warm up. When the butter is hot, pour the eggs and let them cook.

After two minutes, the eggs should be creamy. Add some spinach to your eggs and you can finish scrambling and enjoy!

Keto Recipe #2
Pesto Chicken Casserole
What's in it?

- Peppers
- Some salt
- Chopped garlic cloves (1)
- Diced feta cheese (8 oz.)
- Pitted olives (8 Tbsp.)
- Heavy whip cream (1.5 cups)
- Green pesto (3 oz.)
- Butter (2 oz.)
- Chicken thighs (1.5 lbs.)
- Leafy greens (5.3 oz.)
- Olive oil (4 Tbsp.)

How's it done?

1. Allow the oven to heat up to 400 degrees. While the oven is heating up, cut up the chicken thighs into pieces and season them with pepper and salt.

2. Add the chicken to a skillet and fry them with some butter to make them nice and brown.

3. In another bowl, mix together the heavy cream and the pesto. Place the chicken pieces into a prepared baking dish.

4. Top the chicken with the pesto, garlic, feta cheese, and olives. Place everything into the oven to bake.

5. After 30 minutes, the dish is done and ready to eat.

Keto Recipe #3
Cheese Roll-Ups
What's in it?
- Butter (2 oz.)
- Cheddar cheese (8 oz.)

How's it done?
1. Take the cheese slices onto a cutting board. Slice the butter with a cheese slicer so you end up with thin slices.

2. Cover each of these slices with some butter before rolling them up and then serve and eat.

Keto Recipe #4
Chicken Soup
What's in it?
- Sliced green cabbage (2 cups)
- Shredded chicken (1.5 lbs.)
- Carrot (1)
- Chicken broth (8 cups)
- Pepper (.25 tsp.)
- Salt (1 tsp.)
- Parsley (2 tsp.)
- Minced onion (2 Tbsp.)
- Garlic cloves (2)
- Mushrooms, sliced (6 oz.)
- Celery stalks (2)
- Butter (4 oz.)

How's it done?
1. Start this out by melting the butter in a pot. Slice up the mushrooms and the celery into small pieces.

2. Add these to a pot along with the garlic and dried onion and cook for a few minutes.

3. After this time, add the pepper, salt, parsley, carrot, and broth. Let it all simmer until they become tender.

4. Add the cabbage and the chicken and cook for about 12 more minutes so the noodles are tender before serving.

Keto Recipe #5
Keto Pizza
What's in it?
- *Crust*
- Shredded cheese (6 oz.)
- Eggs (4)
- *Toppings*
- Salt
- Pepper
- Olive oil (4 Tbsp.)
- Leafy greens (5.5 oz.)
- Olives
- Pepperoni (1.75 oz.)
- Shredded cheese (4.25 oz.)
- Dried oregano (1 tsp.)
- Tomato paste (3 Tbsp.)

How's it done?

1. Allow the oven to heat up to 400 degrees. While the oven warms up, take out a bowl and beat the cheese and eggs together to make the crust. Spread this out on a prepared baking sheet, making one large pizza or two small pizzas.

2. Place the pizza(s) in the oven to bake. After 15 minutes, the crust will be golden and you can take the pizza(s) out of the oven.

3. Allow the temperature of your oven to get to 450 degrees. Spread out the tomato paste on your crust and add on the rest of the toppings.

4. Place the pizza(s) back into the oven for a bit and after ten minutes, the pizza(s) should be ready. Serve with some leafy green vegetables and enjoy.

Keto Recipe #6
Smoked Salmon
What's in it?
- Pepper
- Salt
- Lime (1/2)
- Olive oil (1 Tbsp.)
- Baby spinach (2 oz.)
- Mayo (1 cup)
- Smoked salmon (.75 lbs.)

How's it done?
1. To start, bring out a plate and put the lime wedge, spinach, salmon and some mayo all on one plate.

2. Drizzle a bit of oil on top of the spinach before seasoning with the pepper and the salt. Serve this right away and eat.

Keto Recipe #7
Mushroom Omelet
What's in it?
- Pepper

- Salt
- Mushrooms (3)
- Yellow onion (1/3)
- Shredded cheese (1 oz.)
- Butter (1 oz.)
- Eggs (3)

How's it done?
1. To start this recipe, bring out a mixing bowl and crack the eggs inside. Season the eggs with pepper and salt and continue whisking to make them frothy.

2. Melt some butter in a skillet and then when it is warm, add the egg mixture.

3. When you notice this omelet is firming but is still a bit raw, add the onion, mushrooms, and cheese to the top.

4. Use a spatula to ease around the edges of your omelet so you can fold it in half. Take off the heat and serve.

Keto Recipe #8
Keto Quesadillas
What's in it?
- *Tortillas*
- Salt (1/2 tsp.)
- Coconut flour (1 Tbsp.)
- Ground psyllium husk powder (1.5 tsp.)
- Cream cheese (6 oz.)
- Egg whites (2)
- Eggs (2)
- *Filling*
- Olive oil (1 Tbsp.)
- Leafy greens (1 oz.)
- Shredded cheese (5 oz.)

How's it done?
1. Allow the oven to heat up to 400 degrees. While the oven is heating up, beat together your egg whites and eggs for a few minutes to make them fluffy. Add the cream cheese to your eggs and mix until they are nice and smooth.

2. In another bowl, whisk together the coconut flour, psyllium husk powder, and salt. Next, add these ingredients to your bowl of eggs and cream cheese a little at a time.

3. When the batter is combined, let it sit for a bit so it becomes thick like pancake batter.

4. Place two baking sheets on the counter and add parchment paper. Pour three circles of the dough on each sheet and spread into thin rounds.

5. Next, place the two sheets of dough into the oven and let the dough cook for a bit. After five minutes, you can take the tortillas out.

6. When the tortillas have cooled down, place them onto a cutting board and add some cheese on the tortillas. Also, add on some leafy green vegetables and the rest of the cheese on the tortilla and then top it with a second tortilla.

7. Take out a skillet and add in some oil. Fry each of the quesadillas in the skillet for a bit on each side, letting the cheese melt.

8. After this is done, cut up the quesadillas and then serve and eat.

Keto Recipe #9
Asian Stir-Fry

What's in it?
- Sesame oil (1 Tbsp.)
- Ginger (1 Tbsp.)
- Chili flakes (1 tsp)
- Sliced scallions (3)
- Garlic cloves (2)
- White wine vinegar (1 Tbsp.)
- Pepper (.25 tsp. or 1/4 tsp.)
- Onion powder (1 tsp.)
- Salt (1 tsp.)
- Ground beef (1.5 lbs.)
- Butter (5.5 oz.)
- Green cabbage (1.66 lbs.)
- *Wasabi Mayo*
- Wasabi paste (1 Tbsp.)
- Mayonnaise (1 cup)

How's it done?
1. Shred up the cabbage with your food processor. Add some butter to a frying pan and then fry your cabbage for a few minutes.

2. Add the vinegar and spices and cook for a few more minutes before putting the cabbage in a bowl.

3. Melt the remainder of the butter before adding the ginger, chili flakes, and garlic and then let it cook. Add the meat and let it get brown all the way through.

4. Add the cabbage and the scallions to this mixture and stir to make it hot. Top with sesame oil, pepper, and salt.

5. Before serving, mix the ingredients together with the mayonnaise. Serve this stir-fry with some of the wasabi mayo on top.

Keto Recipe #10
Keto Pancakes
What's in it?
- Butter (2 oz.)
- Ground psyllium husk powder (1 Tbsp.)
- Cottage cheese (7 oz.)
- Eggs (4)
- *Toppings Below*
- Whipping cream (1 cup)
- Fresh berries (8 Tbsp.)

How's it done?
1. To start this recipe, take out a bowl and blend all the batter ingredients together. Set the bowl to the side and let it expand for at least five minutes.

2. When you are ready, heat up a bit of the oil in a pan. Add some of the batter to the pan and let the batter cook for three minutes on both sides. Make sure to flip the batter (pancake) carefully.

3. Turn off the heat when the pancake is done and serve with the heavy cream and the berries of your choice before enjoying your meal.

Chapter 8: The Ketogenic Diet vs. Intermittent Fasting

The ketogenic diet can be a very effective diet plan.

If you are able to eat the right foods and closely monitor your macronutrients, you will enter into ketosis and see big results.

Still, some people hit a rut with their weight loss goals or simply need to do even more to help improve their overall health.

As a result, working with just the ketogenic diet may not be enough for some people.   One diet alternative that people can choose to practice is called intermittent fasting.

What is Intermittent Fasting?

Intermittent fasting is more of a lifestyle than a diet. Intermittent fasting is simply fasting or not eating food for a certain period of time.

Now that period of time of fasting or not eating food is usually between 12-16 hours. However, many people experience better results by fasting for 16 or more hours.

There are a lot of different variations when it comes to intermittent fasting, so you can choose the method that works the best for your schedule or for you to maintain for the long term.

Let's take a look at some of the basics of intermittent fasting so you can see how it will work well with the ketogenic diet.

The Intermittent Fasting Approach

There are actually a few different approaches that you can use when it comes to intermittent fasting.

Each intermittent fasting approach can be effective, and it is often based on what
fits your schedule.

The most common approaches that you can use with intermittent fasting are:

- **Skipping meals:** With this option, you will skip over a meal or two so that you can induce some extra time for fasting.

  So, for example, skipping breakfast or simply not eating in the morning can be one intermittent fasting approach.

  Skipping breakfast is one of the most effective methods for practicing intermittent fasting simply because you are already fasting all night from you last meal (dinner).

  If you must eat breakfast every morning than maybe try to skip either lunch and simply eat dinner.

  The benefit of this intermittent fasting approach is that it allows you to experiment to see what works for you and your schedule.

- **Eating windows:** With this intermittent fasting approach, you are going to work on getting all of your macronutrients within a certain eating schedule.

  For example, a person can have an eating window from 12:00 PM-7:00 PM. So, this means a person can eat from 12:00 PM – 7:00 PM.

  So, while most people eat from when they get up until when they go to bed, a personal practicing this intermittent fasting approach will reduce their eating time to windows of four to eight hours depending on their work and lifestyle schedules.

For example, you can have an eating window from 8:00 AM – 4:00 PM. So, this means you can only eat between 8:00 AM – 4:00 PM.

So, within this eating window you can eat two or three small meals. This intermittent fasting approach is good because you can experiment to see what is convenient for your work and lifestyle schedules.

- **One to two-day cleanses:** With this intermittent fasting approach, you are going to put yourself on an extended fasting period.

  With one to two-day cleanses, you will simply avoid eating for one or two days. You can do one or two-day cleanses once or twice a week.

  Now this intermittent fasting approach will effectively reduce the number of calories that you consume resulting in great weight loss.

  Most people will find that it is hard to start out with a one or two day fast, which is why restricting your eating window or skipping meals are two of the best intermittent fasting approaches you can choose from.

  Remember to experiment with intermittent fasting and try out different eating windows for a week or so to see what intermittent fasting approach works best for you.

How Does Intermittent Fasting Work?

While there are a few different options when it comes to choosing an intermittent fasting approach, you may wonder why it can be so effective.

The whole point of intermittent fasting is to simply eat food during a certain period of time.

Our bodies will only be able to take in so much food at once, so if we are only allowed to eat for a few hours during the day and then fast during the rest, we are limiting our calorie intake which results in weight loss.

During the fasting time, we are not allowed to eat at all. Our metabolism also seems to speed up as long as the fasting period is short, such as fasting for just eighteen hours rather than for a whole week or more.

So not only are we reducing the calories that we are able to consume because our bodies can't take in that much food at one time, we are also speeding up our metabolism at the same time.

Over time, your body is going to learn how to adjust to intermittent fasting.

In the beginning, intermittent fasting is going to be hard and you may feel hungry during the fasting period.

But if you can maintain your periods of fasting, the body will eventually adapt and you will be able to feel just fine without eating all day long.

In addition, maintaining your periods of fasting and keeping track of the food you eat will eventually become easier when you only have a few hours a day to eat.

It is important to state that when you are in a fasting state, the body is able to break down some of the extra fat that is being stored by your body.

Now if you include ketosis from the ketogenic diet, all of the excess fat that you have on your body will simply melt off in no time.

In addition, you will still have plenty of energy for all of your daily activities.

Ketosis actually mimics the fasting state because we take the glucose out of our bloodstream so that we can use fats as our main source of energy.

During your fast, the body is going to rely on those extra fat stores to help you to stay energized.

If you are doing intermittent fasting along with the ketogenic diet, you need to make sure that you really get the sufficient amount of fat content that the body needs so that the body can get the right amounts of energy that it needs.

It is important to state that when you combine both intermittent fasting and the ketogenic diet together, you will be able to burn through fat, lower your glucose levels, and see tremendous results in your overall health.

Intermittent fasting is not necessarily for weight loss, although it can help you to lose weight if you are prone to overeating throughout the day.

In addition, intermittent fasting can help you reduce your calorie intake resulting in weight loss.

When you combine intermittent fasting with the ketogenic diet, you are sure to see some tremendous weight loss results as well as an increase in your health benefits.

Are the Ketogenic Diet and Intermittent Fasting Similar?

There are a few similarities that you will find with the ketogenic diet and intermittent fasting.

Both are going to work to limit the amount of glucose in your diet so that the body will start to rely more on using fats for energy rather than carbs and sugars for energy.

This is an effective way to melt the fat off your body and help you to lose weight.

However, the methods that both use to help you reach this result are different. The ketogenic diet helps you to use fat as energy by changing up the macronutrients that you consume to cut out the carbs.

Intermittent fasting will help you to burn fat because you will be forced to reduce how many calories you are able to consume as a result of having a small eating window.

The ketogenic diet is an eating plan. With the ketogenic diet you have certain foods that you are able to consume, and you need to stick with eating those specific foods if you want to be on this diet plan.

On the other hand, intermittent fasting can be done with any type of diet plan. However, intermittent fasting will not be effective if you only eat junk food during your eating window.

But you can combine intermittent fasting with other diets such as the Mediterranean diet, or any other diet plan that you choose.

But when intermittent fasting is combined with the ketogenic diet, you are going to get some amazing weight loss results and your overall health will greatly improve.

Can I Use Intermittent Fasting and the Ketogenic Diet Together?

Yes, it is possible to use both intermittent fasting and the ketogenic diet together.

Keep in mind, intermittent fasting is more about fasting or not eating for a certain period of time each and every day and that period of time can be between 12-16 hours or more.

Now the ketogenic diet is more about the types of foods that you would eat each and every day specifically low carbs, a lot of healthy fats and moderate protein.

It is important to state that you do not have to go on an intermittent fasting diet in order to lose weight with the ketogenic diet.

It is already hard enough for many people to follow the ketogenic diet so combining both intermittent fasting and the ketogenic diet for weight loss is not required, but instead an option.

But for those people who would like to experiment and seek to achieve their weight loss goals and improve their overall health, then combining both intermittent fasting and the ketogenic diet is definitely a great idea.

With intermittent fasting, you will limit the hours that you are able to eat. Instead of allowing yourself to spread your meals and your snacks all throughout the day, you will limit your "eating window" to just a few hours a day.

With intermittent fasting, many people will choose to only eat between 10:00 AM - 6:00 PM and eat all of their macronutrients during this time period.

Others will do a whole day of fasting once or twice a week where they are not allowed to eat at all for one full day.

When people do a full day of fasting they try to consume all of their nutrients on the other days of the week in order to have sufficient energy for their one full day of fasting.

Just keep in mind that the point of intermittent fasting is that you are limiting the amount of time that you are able to eat which forces you to eat fewer calories which results in weight loss.

Now if you ever feel like you hit a plateau with your weight loss goals while on the ketogenic diet, simply consider combining the ketogenic diet with intermittent fasting.

Combining both the ketogenic diet and intermittent fasting will definitely "shock" the body and you will also benefit greatly by burning more fat and achieving your weight loss goals.

When you combine intermittent fasting with the ketogenic diet, you must remember to stick with the macronutrients that we discussed above that are approved for the ketogenic diet.

So, you will still stick with a high fat, moderate protein, and low carb diet plan even while intermittent fasting.

You will just need to be more careful about the times you eat those macronutrients, but otherwise, you can follow the ketogenic diet exactly the same.

If you want to get some of the benefits that come with intermittent fasting or you want to increase your weight loss, then combining intermittent fasting with the ketogenic diet can be very effective.

You can experiment with the different types of intermittent fasting variations that are available to see which one fits into your schedule and works best for you.

Of course, if you find the ketogenic diet is effective enough or adding in intermittent fasting is too difficult, you can always just stay with the ketogenic diet on its own and still see some amazing results.

Conclusion

Thank you for making it through the end of this book.

I hope the book was educational, informative and able to provide you with all of the tools you need to achieve your health and weight loss goals or whatever they may be.

The next step is to get started with the ketogenic diet.

This is one of the most effective diet plans that is available for helping you to lose weight.

While you will need to get used to some of the dietary changes that are unusual compared to other traditional diet plans, the ketogenic diet will really help you to lose weight in no time.

So, what you have come to learn from this book is what exactly the ketogenic diet is all about and how you can use it for your own weight loss journey.

You have learned the basics of the ketogenic diet, the benefits of trying it out, how you can use it with intermittent fasting to lose more weight, the foods that are allowed on the ketogenic diet, and even some meal plans to help you get started.

It is important to mention that the more information that you have before starting the ketogenic diet, the more you will be successful with this diet.

Just keep in mind that when you are tired of trying out all the other diet plans that haven't been successful in the past and you want to work with something that will actually work, the ketogenic diet is always a great option for weight loss.

Thanks again for choosing to read my book and I wish you great success with the ketogenic diet.

31 Ideas for Successfully Burning Fat

Below are 31 of the Best Ideas for Burning Fat.

#1 Develop a Health and Fitness Chief Aim

*Use the following guide for achieving your health and fitness goals.

Step #1
Write down your health and fitness goal(s) and be specific. For example, if you want to lose 10 pounds then write down, "I want to lose 10 pounds."

At the same time, if you want to build muscle, be specific and write down the amount of muscle you want to have. For example, if you want to have 10 pounds of muscle then write down, "I want to have 10 pounds of muscle."

Step #2
Write down the date by which you want to achieve your health and fitness goal(s).

For example, "I will lose 10 pounds by February 2019."

Example two, "I will be able to run 15 miles nonstop by May 2019."

Step 3

Write down what you are willing to sacrifice in order to achieve your health and fitness goals. In addition, write down what are you willing to give back (to the world) in return for achieving your health and fitness goal(s).

For example, "I am willing to give up drinking alcohol, specifically beer for the next 3 months in order to lose 20 pounds of fat. In addition, I am going to stop watching television after 10:00 PM and I will instead go to sleep early so that I can wake up early and exercise."

"In return for achieving my health and fitness goals, I will serve as a role model inspiring and helping others to also achieve their health and fitness goals by sharing my knowledge, experience and wisdom."

Step 4
Repeat looking and reading over your Health and Fitness Chief Aim every day until you achieve your health and fitness goals. In addition, look and read over your Health and Fitness Chief Aim multiple times a day. Daily repetition is important for achieving any goal.

#2 Learn to Cook Healthy Food in Under 20 minutes

Believe it or not but you can learn to cook healthy food in under 20 minutes!

In order to cook healthy food in under 20 minutes it is important to follow the **Kiss Principal** which stands for:

K=Keep
I=It

S=Simple
S=Stupid

Here are four great, easy to make recipes that you can use for cooking healthy food in under 20 minutes:

Recipe 1 (Chicken Fajitas)

- Chop chicken breast into small pieces and cook high on a pan for 10-15 minutes.
- Serve chopped chicken with precooked sweet potatoes that are reheated.
- Include a large bowl of washed lettuce with your meal.
  *Add some low sodium hot sauce to your Chicken Fajitas for some spicy flavor.

Recipe 2 (Breakfast/Lunch Oats)

- Use Sugar Free Oatmeal or Steel Cut Oats.
- Boil Hot Water for 5-10 Minutes.
- Pour hot water onto bowl of oatmeal and stir for 2 or 3 minutes.
- Serve Oatmeal with Frozen Greek Yogurt.
  *Add blueberries, almonds or cashews to your Oatmeal

Recipes 3 (Scrambled Eggs with Avocado)

1. Cook 3 or 4 whole scrambled eggs.
2. Serve eggs with 1 large avocado (feel free to mix avocado with eggs).

3. Include a large bowl of washed spinach with your meal.

    *Desert can be some blackberries, walnuts and dark chocolate

Recipe 4 (Fish and Veggies)

- Open 1 or 2 cans of tuna.

- Serve with low sodium whole wheat crackers.

- Include frozen mixed veggies or spinach.

    *Add some low sodium sauce to your tuna.

#3 Cook For 2 or 3 Days!

When you cook, consider cooking enough healthy food to last you 2 or 3 days.

Cooking enough food to last you 2 or 3 days will definitely save you a lot of time!

Consider cooking simple foods like chicken breasts, which can be cooked in under 20 minutes and save the leftovers in the refrigerator.

You can also boil multiple sweet potatoes while at home and save any leftovers in the fridge.

What is great about boiling sweet potatoes is that they are extremely healthy for you and they involve No Cooking whatsoever!

Cooking enough healthy food to last you 2 or 3 days is a great way to make sure you always have something healthy to eat no matter how busy you are.

In addition, cooking enough food that last you 2 or 3 days is a great way to cut down on the amount of time you spend cooking and cleaning in the kitchen.

#4 Order Your Groceries from The Internet

If you hate going to a crowded supermarket or your simply just too busy to go grocery shopping then consider shopping for groceries online!

Here are some advantages of shopping for groceries online:

Convenience: You don't have to wait in long lines to purchase your groceries. Instead, you can do your grocery shopping online in minutes. Plus, you can shop for your groceries 24 hours a day, 7 days a week!

Better Prices: You can sometimes get better prices from online grocery stores because they want more and more people to use their services.

In addition, some online grocery stores may even offer coupons and free home delivery.

Fewer Expenses: You don't have to pay for gas for your car when you shop for groceries online.

You don't even need to own a car to shop online! Instead you can simply save money by not having a car and by simply shopping for your groceries online and having them delivered directly to your home.

Delivery to Your Front Door: You don't have to worry about going out in the snow, rain or during busy rush hour traffic to purchase groceries.

You can instead simply order your groceries online and simply have them delivered to your home for a small free and sometimes for free!

No Unwanted Unhealthy Food: It's far too easy to walk into a supermarket and be tempted to buy unhealthy food.

Instead, buying groceries online simply allows you to buy exactly what you need without having any temptations to purchase additional foods especially all those delicious looking deserts that are usually placed at the entrance of supermarkets.

#5 Use The 80/20 Rule

The 80/20 Rule is a very simple principle that goes like this: 80% of the time eat healthy and 20% of the time eat whatever you want and this could include your favorite dessert.

For example, let's say you eat a healthy dinner that consists of skinless chicken breasts, boiled sweet potatoes and a bowl of spinach.

If you decide to include a small bowl of chocolate ice-cream then you now just made dessert part of your dinner.

So, around 80% of your dinner consisted of healthy foods such as chicken breasts, sweet potatoes and spinach and the other 20% consisted of your chocolate ice-cream dessert which is not considered a top healthy food choice.

If you apply the 80/20 Rule to your eating habits, you will develop the habit of eating healthy 80% percent of the time while you give yourself some space to enjoy some of your favorite desserts and foods 20% of the time.

#6 Eliminate or Limit Your Alcohol Intake

Plain and simple…alcohol, especially beer makes you fat!

The more beer you drink that fatter you will get. In addition, drinking alcohol especially beer can make you hungry causing you too eat unhealthy fast food.

As a result, limit your alcohol intake or completely eliminate it.

If you are going to drink, consider drinking a small glass of red wine.

#7 Avoid Overeating With "Portion Control"

Overeating can cause weight gain, even if you are eating healthy foods.

However, you can prevent excess weight gain from overeating by practicing "portion control."

"Portion control" is simply reducing the amount of food you eat by eating smaller portions.

The best way to reduce the amount of food you eat is by using a small food scale. You can also consider using a smaller bowl or plate for reducing the amount of food you eat.

However, using a food scale for reducing the amount of food you eat is 100% more accurate than using a small bowl or plate.

When it comes to "portion control" using a food scale, all you have to do is simply weigh your food before you eat it so that you will know exactly how much food you are consuming for each meal.

So, if you want to simply lose a few extra pounds all you have to do is simply reduce the amount of food you are eating by using your food scale.

The concept of "portion control" is very popular with bodybuilders, weightlifters and competitive athletes.

Nutritionists are also known to recommend their clients to use "portion control" as a way of reducing obesity.

#8 Eat Natural Foods

To lose weight, stay healthy and keep your energy levels high as you strive to be a successful in life, it is very important to eat natural foods.

Why eat natural foods?

Because, foods like fruits, vegetables, nuts, lean cuts of meat and healthy fats have a lot of vitamins and minerals that are excellent for providing the body and mind with optimal health.

Here are some more benefits of eating Natural Foods:

- Natural foods will help boost your energy levels for optimal performance giving you superior energy to work harder and smarter.

- Natural foods are great for fighting off chronic diseases and illness as well as for preventing you from getting sick.

- Natural foods like fruits and veggies are low calorie water foods that will supply your body with a lot of water and fiber and will help you to feel full and eat less.

- Because natural foods are healthier for you, they will help you to lose weight.

Keep in mind that the more natural foods you eat, the more weight you will lose.

In addition, you will have more energy, feel healthier and be able to perform at your best as a result of eating more natural foods.

#9 Practice Intermittent Fasting

Intermittent fasting is a very effective healthy eating method that any busy person can incorporate into their busy lives.

Intermittent fasting works by eating within a certain time period or an "eating window" within a day and then fasting for the rest of the day.

For example, let's say you have an "eating window" Monday - Friday from 11:00 AM – 7:00 PM.

This means that you can eat (usually 1 or 2 meals or more) from 11:00 AM – 7:00 PM. Once your "eating window" closes, you simply fast for the rest of the day.

When you temporarily fast for a period of time, you get to experience all kinds of benefits.

Some of The Benefits of Intermittent Fasting Are:

- You develop discipline with your eating habits.

- You will feel very alert and energetic while fasting.

- Increases your life expectancy.

- Helps you to lose weight and hunger.

- Allows you to develop a flexible eating schedule around your busy work/life.

- Allows you to eat only 1 or 2 meals a day giving you more free time to focus on other priorities.

Overall, intermittent fasting is a great tool that any busy person can use for eating healthy and staying fit.

#10: Use A Food Journal

Using a food journal is a great way to keep track of all the food you eat on a daily basis.

All you have to do is simply write down what eat you every day. Make sure to include any snacks, teas, coffee and drinks in your food journal.

Writing down what you eat using a food journal is a great habit to develop. You will come to realize how healthy you are eating as well as all the unhealthy foods you may be eating.

In addition, you can look back at all the food you ate on any given day and determine whether you ate too much.

If you feel like you are simply eating too much or that you want to lose a few pounds, you can use your food journal as a way to see what foods you may want to eat less of.

You can keep track of the food you eat by using notebook, or you can use your computer or you can even use an app.

Using a food journal is great for helping you to keep focused on your diet, helps you to develop good eating habits, provides motivation for achieving your health and fitness goals and it is an efficient way to simply burn fat and lose weight.

At the end of the day, you can refer back to your food journal and ask yourself questions like:

Did I eat a healthy delicious meal?

Did I eat enough fruits and vegetables?

Did I drink enough water?

Did I eat any unhealthy foods or snacks?

Didi I feel extremely full after each meal?

Did I feel energetic or tired as a result of the foods I ate?

#11 Drink Lots of Water Every Day!

Water is great for the body. But did you know that foods such as a fruits and vegetables are not only full of vitamins and minerals, but they are also full of water?

Simply drinking more water and eating more water foods on a daily basis has so many benefits such as:

- Water gives you lots of energy.

- Water is great for your skin.

- Water prevents you from feeling fatigue as a result of dehydration.

- Water helps you to feel full.

- Prevents you from feeling hungry.

- Helps reduce weight loss.

- Is great for your ligaments, tendons and joints. So, water lubricates your body!

Eating more fruits and vegetables on a daily basis is high recommended not only for the vitamins and nutrients they provide but also for the amount of water they provide.

As a result, don't underestimate the power of water!

Water is magical!

#12 Remove All Junk Food from Your Home

Simply, remove all junk food from your home and instead replace these unhealthy foods with healthy snacks.

Some healthy snacks to eat are fruits and healthy nuts like almonds, walnuts and cashews and you can even eat some dark chocolate!

If you are a busy working professional, consider taking healthy snacks to your office instead of buying unhealthy foods and snacks on the way to work.

#13 Take A Break Every Hour

Simply take a break every hour from sitting down and get your body moving.

You can take a break for 10-15 minutes and maybe do some light stretching or you can even do some dynamic stretches like arm and leg circles as well as hip and waist rotations.

You can even do some easy body-weight exercises like push-ups, body-weight squats or lunges to get the blood flowing in your body.

#14 Set A Schedule and Develop Discipline to Stick to It

Some people are morning people and others are night owls. Do whatever works best for you.

However, develop the habit of creating a work, eating and fitness schedule and stick to it so that you can make sure you are living a healthy lifestyle.

In addition, developing a work, eating and fitness schedule will keep you focused on what is important and what you should focus on as well as what your priorities are.

You will also be more organized if you develop a work, eating and fitness schedule and stick to it than if you had no plan whatsoever.

#15 Create a Healthy Environment

Whether you work from home or from your work office, create an environment that is relaxing and enjoyable for you.

You can look into getting some home/office fitness gear such as a work desk to make sure you are moving your body or you can even use a gym chair which provides a total body workout.

You can even consider getting a cycling work station or a under desk treadmill for the purpose of getting some exercise while you work or watch TV at home.

#16 Sleep More

According to research, sleep is more important than nutrition and exercise.

A lack of sleep will reduce your mental and physical performance. In addition, lack of sleep will develop stress in your body causing you to gain weight.

A lack of sleep will also affect your mood and hormones.

As you can see, you want to make sure you sleep as much as possible especially if you want to burn fat effectively.

Sleep is extremely beneficial for being successful in overall life because it will repair your body and mind from all the mental and physical stress you put it through day after day so make sure you are getting lots and lots of sleep.

I will talk more about the importance of sleep and its benefits later.

#17 Plan Your Meals and Eat the Same Meals

Plan your meals ahead. You can also develop the habit of eating the same healthy foods every day both for lunch and dinner.

This keeps shopping for healthy foods easy and it is an efficient way of eating because you will develop the habit of shopping for and cooking the same foods every day.

#18 Use A Food Scale

Use a food scale to weigh your food before you cook it so that you know exactly how much food you will be consuming every day both for lunch and dinner.

By using a food scale, you will be able to keep track of the number of calories you are eating every day.

In addition, you will be more efficient at losing weight because you will not be overeating as a result of keeping track of how much food you eat.

Research shows that 80% of weight loss is all about your diet and what you eat and how much you eat.

So, by weighing your food, you will know if you need to reduce the number of calories you are eating in order to lose weight.

In addition, weighing your food will help you to maintain your desired weight.

#19 Develop a Health and Fitness Calendar

The same way you have appointments, meetings and deadlines for your work and personal life is the same way you should have them also for your health and fitness goals.

Simply develop a schedule on your calendar that allows you to have time for exercise, rest and recreation.

Developing a health and fitness calendar will help you to break away from your daily routine.

Making health and fitness a priority is a great way to make sure you are giving your body and mind a break from all the stress and challenges you face on a daily basis.

In addition, you will feel more energetic, focused and productive as a result of taking the time to exercise and improve your well-being.

You will also have positive energy, a lot of focus and high levels of productivity that will help you to continue to succeed in losing weight and achieving your personal goals.

So, use a calendar and schedule your workouts, schedule your breaks, schedule your yoga classes, schedule your meals, simply prioritize scheduling your health and fitness lifestyle.

#20 Exercise More

Try to squeeze more exercise into your daily life.

Begin your day with an early walking routine.

Consider working out at home if you are really too busy to make it to the gym.

Whatever you do, try to move more throughout the day because you will feel less fatigue then if you just sit down at a desk all day.

Research shows that exercise improves your ability to think better. In addition, exercise will make you happier and feel better.

Here are some other ways that exercise will improve not only your health but also your mind:

- Increases your level of focus.
- Improves your memory.
- Develops discipline and focus.
- Improves your work performance and time management skills.
- Improves your immune system which means you will not get sick as often.
- Gives you more energy to do more especially when it comes to achieving your health and fitness goals and any other personal goals.

As you can see exercise strongly affects how well you will succeed in your overall life.

As a result, develop an exercise plan and stick to it so that you can experience great results in both your health and in overall life.

#21 Eat More Vegetables, Fish and Fruits

Eat healthier to look and feel better. When you look and feel better you will feel more confident in yourself to achieve more in life.

Simply eating lots of fresh vegetables and fruits will give you all the energy you need to succeed in life and with achieving your health and fitness goals.

In addition, you have to include fish in your diet because it is good for the heart, good for the joints, improves your mood, strengthens your immune system, it improves your sleep and more!

It is important to state that people that eat healthy have higher levels of productivity.

In addition, a person's physical work capacity and performance is greatly increased as a result of eating a healthier diet.

If you still don't think that eating healthy is important than consider this: **research shows that the amount of money that you make is a result of your eating habits.**

So, the healthier you eat the more money you are likely to make. However, if you have a poor diet, then you will simply be poor.

#22 Write Down Everything

Write down your financial goals, your fitness goals, your life goals, write down all your goals and try to slowly accomplish them little by little every day.

You will feel better when you see what you are accomplishing every day by writing down what you achieve every day.

In addition, you will have a better understanding of what areas you need to improve on.

You can refer back to your daily accomplishments knowing that you did everything you could to succeed and as a result you will sleep better.

The next day when you wake up, you will wake up energetic, hungry and ready to get started on your daily projects and goals to see how much you can accomplish.

You will eventually develop healthy habits like drinking more water, sleeping more and getting more exercise as you continue to write down your daily goals and reflect on your accomplishments.

You will come to learn how sleeping more, drinking more water and daily exercise are important for accomplishing any goal in life.

You will soon have a full daily schedule prioritizing your health, work and life goals eliminating everything that is unimportant in life.

As you continue to remain focus on your daily schedule, you will succeed at achieving your goals as a result of developing priorities for achieving your health and fitness and other goals.

You will develop a lot more focus in life as a result of writing down your goals.

So, track your weight loss progress and other goals you want to achieve and be aware if things are working or if you need to make some changes.

#23 Use A Fitness Tracker

If you are a busy person that wants to exercise, eat healthy and feel great but needs some motivation to get stared and remain motivated, then consider using a fitness tracker.

What is a Fitness Tracker?

A fitness tracker is a cool looking device that is more like a small computer that you wear around your wrist like a watch.

Fitness trackers can monitor and track your health and fitness related activities like keeping count of your running mileage as well as how many calories you have burned.

Fitness trackers can even monitor your sleep as well as your heart rate and more!

Overall, fitness trackers are great for motivating you to get in shape as well as stay in shape.

Here are some more ways fitness trackers can help you achieve your health and fitness goals:

- Keep track of your daily health and fitness progress.
- Provide free workouts and tips.
- Help you set achievable fitness goals.
- Monitor your sleep patterns and breathing.
- Assist you with developing healthy habits like walking more and eating less.
- Send alerts to remind you to get up and move more.
- Monitors your diet, calories, and the foods you eat.
- Assists with training for a marathon and burning fat.

What is great about fitness trackers is that they act like a personal trainer that is always conveniently available to you 24 hours a day, 7 days a week, 365 days a year.

Overall, fitness trackers are one of the best ways to make sure you achieve your health and fitness goals.

#24 Use A Fitness App

Research show that people that use fitness apps are likelier to remain consistent with their health and fitness lifestyle then people that don't use fitness apps.

In addition, research also shows that people that use fitness apps are more active than people that don't use fitness apps.

As you can see, fitness apps are great for keeping you in shape. In addition, there are all kinds of fitness apps that you can use from running apps to strength training apps to yoga apps to even nutrition apps.

Overall, fitness apps are great for making sure you stay consistent with your health and fitness lifestyle.

#25 Make A Commitment to Exercise

It is important to be consistent with getting some exercise every day no matter how busy you may be.

Simply, don't make excuses for not be able to exercise whether you are busy at work, with your family or if you have something else going on.

In addition, don't make excuses that you can't exercise because you are sick or tired or the weather is too cold or it is raining outside.

Instead do whatever it takes to get some exercise every day and that can be from running outside to doing some bodyweight exercises at home.

No matter what, have a fitness plan and be consistent with your training schedule.

#26 Do Full Body Workouts

To make sure you burn the most amount of calories, focus on exercising your entire body by doing full body workouts.

Full body workouts are great because you will exercise the entire body in a short amount of time and burn a lot of calories.

Here are some circuit routines for a Full Body Workout:

<u>Circuit Routine 1 (4-6 Sets)</u>

- Bodyweight squats (12-15) repetitions
- Pushups (8-12) repetitions
- Sit-ups (10-15) repetitions

  *rest 1 minute

<u>Circuit Routine 2 (4-6 Sets)</u>

- Lunges (alternate forward and reverse) (12-15) repetitions
- Diamond Pushups (8-12) repetitions

- Bodyweight planks (30-45 seconds)

  *rest 1 minute

<u>Circuit Routine 3 (4-6 Sets)</u>
- Pushup Burpees (6-8) repetitions
- Flutter kicks (12-15) repetitions
- Mountain climbers (10-12) repetitions

  *rest 1 minute

#27 Keep Track of Your Fitness Goals

Keep track of your health and fitness goals day after day, week after week, month after month.

You can do so by writing down your workouts and your progress. In addition, keep a food journal.

Try to write down what you ate and what time you ate especially if you are practicing the ketogenic diet or intermittent fasting or both.

#28 Prioritize Your Diet

Although exercise is great for the body, mind and spirit, when it comes to losing weight, it is all about your DIET.

Simply to be lean and stay in shape you really have to focus on your diet.

So, if you can really focus on your diet in addition to getting some daily exercise, you will be able to remain fit 365 days a year.

To make sure you are staying in shape day after day, week after week, month after month make every attempt to eat a lot of vegetables, nuts, lean meats and fruits.

You can also consider shopping at the local farmer's market to make sure that the food you are buying is fresh.

#29 Do Some Exercise Early in The Morning

If you want to make sure you exercise every day, then simply try to go to sleep a little earlier so that you can wake up a little earlier to get a morning workout.

No matter how buys you may be, it is a good idea to wake up early and do some exercise immediately upon waking up.

Research shows that doing some form of light exercise upon waking up is a great way to get the body and mind ready for the day.

Your morning workout does not have to be long.

You can do a short, intense bodyweight circuit routine or you can simply go for a short 20-minute run or a 30-minute walk.

The point is you want to start your day by being active because later in the day you may get a little lazy and decide not to do any exercise especially if you feel tired.

#30 Use A Standing Desk

A standing desk is a desk that is designed for a person to use while standing up.

A person can use a standing desk to comfortably read, write or do some work on a computer or laptop while standing up.

Research shows that you burn more calories when using a standing desk then when you sit down and use a traditional desk.

Simply, when you are standing up, your body is using more energy to remain standing versus when you sit down.

When you are sitting down at a traditional desk, all of your weight is being supported by a chair and many times that chair may not even be comfortable.

In addition, standing desks get you moving around more as well as walking around more because you are more motivated to walk or move around then if you sit down at a traditional desk which simply makes the body and mind too comfortable and lazy.

#31 Sleep Benefits for Weight Loss

Every busy person has a shortage of time. However, when it comes to sleep, a person must make time for getting enough sleep in order to succeed in overall life.

There are so many benefits to exercise and having a healthy diet. But when it truly comes to weight loss, sleep is the secret to fat loss.

Here are 8 reasons why sleep will help you to lose weight:

#1 Sleep Controls Your Diet and Fitness Lifestyle

Believe it or not but sleep is more important than diet and exercise.

The reason why sleep is more important than diet and exercise is because if you don't get enough sleep (7-9 hours) every night, your lack of sleep will negatively affect both your diet and your fitness goals.

Research shows that the more you sleep the more weight you lose because you will have the energy and focus to stick to your diet as well as to exercise with tremendous energy.

This concept of sleeping more to lose more weight is very simple yet very difficult to follow by many people especially busy people.

The solution is to make sleep a priority just like accomplishing your work, family and financial goals are a priority.

#2 Sleep Eliminates Food Cravings

Research shows that getting enough sleep eliminates food cravings because your body is not stressed from a lack of a good night's sleep.

However, when you don't get enough sleep, you cause your body to develop stress.

When you are stressed, this hormone called cortisol causes you to crave food especially unhealthy foods and what happens is that eventually you give in and begin to eat more and more.

Cortisol is responsible for weight gain so whenever your body produces cortisol, you will simply gain weight.

In order to prevent cortisol from developing in the body, you have to make sure you are getting enough sleep.

It does not matter how much you exercise or how strict your diet is. If you do not get enough sleep, your body will be craving food as a result of the stress it undergoes as a result of not getting enough sleep.

#3 Good Quality Sleep Builds Muscle

If you strength train and get a good night's sleep you allow your body to repair itself. In addition, you allow your body to build muscle as a result of getting a good night's sleep.

Building muscle is good for fighting fat because even if you have small amounts of muscle, this muscle will force your body to burn off calories.

#4 Sleep Is the Fountain of Youth

Whenever you get a good night's rest, your body develops Human Growth Hormone (HGH).

Human growth Hormone is a natural hormone that your body develops and is responsible for anti-aging.

More specifically, Human Growth Hormone enhances weight loss, develops stronger bones, builds muscle, reduces cardiovascular disease, improves your mood as well as your cognitive function.

Therefore, the more you sleep, the more Human Growth Hormone your body will develop.

As a result of developing more Human Growth Hormone, you will live longer and feel more youthful and energetic as a result of sleeping more.

#5 Sleep Gives You Superior Energy

When you get a good night of sleep, you wake up feeling refreshed ready to take on the world.

In addition, you will be more motivated to exercise, eat healthy and accomplish your daily goals as a result of getting a good night's sleep.

It is also important to state that getting a good night's sleep will give you razor sharp focus and a strong willingness to accomplish your daily goals.

#6 The More You Sleep the Less You Eat

Research shows that the earlier you go to sleep and the more you sleep (7-9 hours), the less likely you are to eat because you will be eliminating late night snacking and boredom from staying up late.

In addition, sleeping more will help to keep you focused on your diet and health and fitness lifestyle as a result of being well rested.

#7 Sleeping More Burns More Calories

Research shows that you burn more calories when you sleep between 7-9 hours per night then if you were to sleep between 4-6 hours per night.

The reason being is because when you sleep 7-9 hour per night, your body is working more efficiently at burning calories as a result of it being well rested.

However, if you only sleep between 4-6 hours per night, your body will be under tremendous stress and will feel lethargic making your body to burn less calories over time.

#8 A Good Night Sleep Will Help You to Shop for Healthy Foods

Research shows that people that get a good night's rest are likelier to eat healthier as well as shop for healthier food versus people that don't get enough sleep.

This is because people that don't get enough sleep tend to drink sugary drinks like coffee with extra sugar and energy drinks in order to stay awake.

In addition, a person that does not get a good night's rest will be stressed out and will be searching for comfort foods which most likely will be unhealthy foods.

Here are Some Tips for a Better Night's Sleep

- Turn off your computer, cell phone, and TV at least 30 minutes before you go to sleep.

- Make your bed and bedroom as relaxing as possible in order to ensure a good night's sleep.

- Create a nightly bedtime ritual. Consider taking a warm bath or reading a book before going to bed. In addition, eliminate doing any important work before going to bed.

- Develop a bedtime schedule. Figure out what time you want to wake up in the morning then decide to go to sleep every night at the same time making sure you sleep between 7-9 hours every night.

- Eliminate drinking any fluids before you go to sleep in order to prevent waking up at night to go to the toilet. In addition, eliminate drinking coffee early in the evening and stay away from energy drinks, soda and alcohol if possible.

- Try to sleep in complete darkness if possible. If this is uncomfortable consider buying a lamp with a timer that shuts off after a few minutes.

Summary

I hope you enjoyed the **31 Ideas for Successfully Burning Fat**.
.

To get the most out of this entire book, it is important for you to be persistent with achieving your health and fitness goals.

In addition, it is important to develop resilience and persevere when confronted with challenges along your health and fitness journey.

Learn to realize that every day, you should have a short list of your top three or four priorities in your life and exercise and living a health and fitness lifestyle should be one of them.

Nevertheless, take what you have learned from this book and apply it to your health and fitness lifestyle.

It can be stated that exercise and living a health and fitness lifestyle is one of the most important habits to have in life.

In addition, the power of exercise and living a health and fitness lifestyle can transform your body, mind and your overall life so embrace it with everything you got.

Bonus

Please continue reading on the following page to access the book,

Intermittent Fasting: The Smart Way to Losing Weight.

INTERMITTENT FASTING

The Smart Way to Losing Weight

by
Epic Rios

"Find an excellent health and fitness habit that you like and slowly let it override any bad habit you want to get rid of." — **E. Rios**

Table of Contents

There are no scenarios in which the publisher or the original author of this work can be in any fashion deemed liable for any hardship or damages that may befall them after undertaking information described herein.

Additionally, the information found on the following pages is intended for informational purposes only and should thus be considered, universal.

As befitting its nature, the information presented is without assurance regarding its continued validity or interim quality.

Trademarks that mentioned are done without written consent and can in no way be considered an endorsement from the trademark holder.

Introduction

Intermittent fasting has grown in popularity in recent years, thanks in large part to its ability to promote greater rates of weight loss compared to other eating methods.

Intermittent fasting has also grown in popularity because it doesn't require radical changes to the types of foods you are eating, when you eat or even drastically alter the number of calories you consume in a 24-hour period.

In fact, the most common type of intermittent fasting approach is to simply consume two slightly larger than average meals during a day instead of the usual three meals a day.

Eating two meals a day makes the intermittent fasting lifestyle an ideal choice for those who find they have difficulty sticking to more stringent diet plans, as it only requires changing one habit, the number of meals per day, instead of many habits all at once.

Many people find that practicing intermittent fasting leads to genuine and sustainable results.

Intermittent fasting is simple enough to manage successfully over a prolonged period of time. Intermittent fasting most definitely provides the type of results that can keep motivation levels high enough once the novelty of the new diet begins to fade.

The secret to intermittent fasting's success is the simple fact that your body behaves differently when it's in a "fasting state" versus a "fed state."

When your body is in what is known as a "fed state," it is actively digesting and absorbing food.

This process of digesting and absorbing food begins some five minutes after you have finished putting food into your body and can last anywhere from three to five hours depending on the how much food you ate as well as what kind of food you ate.

So, for example, if you drink a veggie smoothie then your body will quickly absorb and digest the smoothie because vegetables are very easy for the body to breakdown and digest.

However, if you eat steak or beef, then your body will require more time to absorb and digest the food and this process can last several hours.

It is important to state that while your body is in the "fed state," your body is actively producing insulin which in turn makes it harder for your body to burn fat properly.

After the period of digestion has occurred, insulin levels start dropping back towards normal which can take anywhere from 8 to 12 hours and is the buffer between the "fed and fasted state."

Once your insulin levels return to normal, the "fasted state" begins which is the period where your body begins the process of burning fat more effectively.

Unfortunately, this means that many people never reach the point where they can burn fat most efficiently, as they rarely go eight hours, much less 12 hours from some type of caloric consumption or simply eating.

But, there is hope! To see results with intermittent fasting, all you need to do is simply break the habit of eating three meals a day and this book will teach you how to do so.

Every effort was made to ensure this book is full of as much useful information as possible. Please enjoy!

Chapter 1: How Intermittent Fasting Works

History of Intermittent Fasting

Fasting is not a trend but instead has been a part of some religious practices including Buddhism, Islam, and Christianity for many years.

Even before certain religions began to practice intermittent fasting, it was already known that people that lived many centuries ago used to practice intermittent fasting as a result of the unavailability of food resources.

Just remember, intermittent fasting is not a starvation diet since starvation is considered an involuntary absence of food.

Consider breakfast which is considered a very important time of day for many people.

If you think about the word "breakfast" it translates to "break-fast" which means to break your fast of not eating food all night long.

Fasting dates to the day of Hippocrates of Cos {c460 – c370BC} who is considered in many ideals as the father of modern medicine.

Hippocrates stated, "To eat when you are sick is to feed your illness."

Plato, an ancient Greek thinker, and Aristotle, his student, were great believers and supporters of fasting.

The Greeks believed that fasting is the "physician within." This is the same logic/instinct portrayed by pets.

For example, when a dog is sick it will not eat nor will it force itself to eat but instead it will "fast" until it feels better.

Ben Franklin, an important founding father of America, also stated, "The best of all medicine is resting and fasting."

Intermittent Fasting - The Basics

Intermittent fasting is a way of eating to ensure that you get the most out of every meal you eat.

The core tenants of intermittent fasting mean that you don't need to change what you are eating. Instead, you must change "when" you eat.

However, it is always a great idea to try to eat as healthy as possible and disregard unhealthy foods.

It is important to state that intermittent fasting is a viable alternative to traditional diets because it will help people that "fast" lean up without changing the number of calories they consume in a day.

In fact, the preferred method of intermittent fasting is to simply eat two large meals every day instead of three (or more) meals a day.

Intermittent fasting is also a great option for those who traditionally have trouble sticking to diet plans since intermittent fasting only requires you to change one small habit, instead of several larger habits.

Intermittent fasting is extremely effective for most people because it is simple enough for people to try it out.

And for those individuals who do try intermittent fasting, they will quickly come to realize all of its benefits.

The key to understating why intermittent fasting is so successful lies in the differences in your body during a "fasted state" versus a "fed state."

In addition, intermittent fasting is so effective because of simply changing your eating habits and sticking with them.

The body is considered to be in the "fed state" when it is in the process of absorbing and digesting food.

The "fed state" tends to start roughly five minutes after you begin eating, and lasting from three to five hours, depending on how long it takes your body to digest your meal.

A "fed state," in turn, leads to higher levels of insulin which makes it a lot more difficult for the body to burn fat.

The period directly after the "fed sate" is referred to as the "post-absorptive state" which is the period of time where the body is not actively processing food and the body's insulin
levels begin to fall.

The "post-absorptive state" lasts between eight and twelve hours and directly precedes the "fasted state."

The "fasted state" occurs between nine and twelve hours after the "post-absorptive state" and is the point where the body's insulin levels are at its lowest which in turn make it the period of time where the most fat can be burned during physical activity.

Unfortunately for many people, they rarely go twelve hours without eating which means that no matter how hard they exercise they are not burning fat as efficiently as possible.

However, if you do "fast" beyond twelve hours this also means that you can burn fat and build muscle by simply altering your eating habits.

Scientific Proof

Your metabolic rate is increased with short-term fasting because of the hormonal changes that occur in your body as a result of intermittent fasting.

Studies have shown that weight loss occurs after three to twenty-four weeks on an intermittent fasting program.

In addition, studies have shown that weight loss is not temporary but instead maintained as long as a person continues to live an intermittent fasting lifestyle.

In comparison to other studies that have been done on weight loss, researchers have concluded that intermittent fasting is most certainly effective for weight loss.

In other studies that have been done on intermittent fasting, researchers discovered that many of the individuals that had been on an intermittent fasting program lost 4.0 to 7.0% of his/her waist circumference.

Researchers determined that intermittent fasting is effective for weight loss and that any harmful buildup of belly fat can cause disease and other issues around the body's organs.

One thing to keep in mind is that any results of weight loss from intermittent fasting result from eating fewer overall calories.

In addition, it is important to maintain a sensible eating diet and not indulge in any binge eating while practicing intermittent fasting.

While the science behind intermittent fasting is certainly promising, there are a few things you will need to keep in mind when starting any new dietary plan.

No diet, regardless of how miraculous it appears, can help you if you don't follow a few golden rules:

- *Keep a calorie deficit:* While this is true for any diet, it is even more true for intermittent fasting.

  Since you will limit the number of meals you eat in a day, it can be very easy to overeat once you do eat.

  So, simply eat naturally as you would with any other meal without having the feeling that you have to eat more in order to remain full.

  (Keep this in mind when losing weight: you need to burn 3,500 calories a week to lose one pound of fat each week.)

- *Maintain self-control:* Intermittent fasting only works if your body goes completely without food for at least twelve hours and any caloric intake no matter how small will break the fasting cycle.

  As a result, it is extremely important to make sure that you maintain complete control of your urges to eat snacks or consume soft drinks while practicing intermittent fasting.

  Simply, if you hope to see real results from intermittent fasting, you have to be disciplined and have self-control.

Remember, fasting for at least twelve hours only allows you to eat normally or slightly more than an average meal.

So, keep in mind, fasting for at least twelve hours a day does not give you the license to eat everything in sight.

Remember, keeping your appetite in check is a strict requirement for success while practicing intermittent fasting.

- *Be consistent:* Regardless of the type of diet or weight loss approach that you ultimately choose to pursue, it is important to choose one and stick with it.

  Attempting to do an intermittent fast for a few days before switching to another diet plan such as the Paleo diet before trying out a low-carb approach will only cause your body to freak out and hold on to every possible calorie until it figures out what in the world you are trying to do.

  Remember, practicing intermittent fasting regularly and consistently is the surest way to see any of its real benefits.

  In addition, only after your body has time to adjust to your new intermittent fasting lifestyle will it then be able to adapt to the fasting lifestyle appropriately.

  It is important to state that as you continue to practice intermittent fasting, the body will begin to increase several positive enzymes and neural pathways in order to maximize weight loss.

Before moving on, keep this in mind when practicing intermittent fasting – **be consistent with your intermittent fasting approach.**

If you are consistent with your intermittent fasting approach than you will greatly succeed with losing weight.

So, consistency is the key to success when it comes to losing weight with intermittent fasting.

Possible Side Effects of Intermittent Fasting

While intermittent fasting has some scientifically proven benefits, it is not with its potential side effects.

The biggest side effect of intermittent fasting is the initial change in your bowel movements as periods of constipation or in some cases diarrhea may occur.

Fortunately, periods of constipation or diarrhea should not last more than a few days as your body adjusts to the new intermittent fasting lifestyle.

However, additional side effects can occur to the body if periods of fasting are routinely followed by periods of excessive binge eating.

It is important to begin intermittent fasting slowly and in moderation.

For example, you can begin practicing intermittent fasting by first doing it for one day a week.

Then the following week you can increase it to two days a week and so on until you feel comfortable practicing intermittent fasting every day.

Keep in mind that if you experience any serious immediate physical changes after you begin intermittent fasting simply stop fasting and consult a doctor.

Chapter 2: Various Intermittent Approaches and Fasting Schedules

While the core ideas behind the various forms of intermittent fasting are all the same, there are quite a few different ways to go about it.

Your best bet is to try a few different intermittent fasting approaches and see which one your body naturally responds to the best as well as which approach is convenient for you.

(16 Hours of Fasting: 8 Hour Eating Window) Intermittent Fasting Method

This method involves fasting for 16 hours for men, or 14 hours for women, and then having a window to eat for the next 8 hours for men and 10 hours for women.

A window of eating simply means that you can only eat between certain hours.

For example, your eating window can be from 12:00 PM – 8:00 PM, or 11:00 AM – 7:00 PM or 9:00 AM – 5:00 PM.

Your eating window simply depends on your fasting schedule and what is convenient for you.

So, let's say you have an eating window from 12:00 PM – 8:00 PM.

So, at 12:00 PM you will break your "fast" and eat lunch. Then, maybe at 3:30 PM you eat a small healthy snack.

Then at around 7:30 PM you eat dinner and finish around 8:00 PM.

So, as you can see from this example your eating window is from 12:00 PM – 8:00 PM.

It is important to keep in mind that while you are fasting for 16 hours, you should not eat any food at all during these fasting hours.

You should only consume items that have zero calories including black coffee, water and sugar-free gum.

The easiest way to attempt this intermittent fasting approach (**16 hours of fasting and 8-hour eating window**) is to stop eating after dinner in the evening and then fast for 16 hours or more.

For example, if you finish eating dinner at 7:00 PM then you will begin fasting from 7:00 PM until 11:00 AM the following day.

So, after 11:00 AM, you can break your "fast" and begin eating.

It is important to state that the specifics of when you fast or what time you begin to fast are not nearly as important as ensuring that you fast at the same time regularly every day.

If you often vary the time you fast every day, it can lead to an erratic change in your hormones, which among other things, makes it more difficult for your body to shed any excess weight.

For example, if Monday you begin to fast at 6:00 PM then on Tuesday you begin to fast at 9:00 PM then on Wednesday you begin to fast at 7:00 PM, well your body may find it hard to adapt to your fasting schedule.

As a result, you may end up breaking your fast and eat because you are not consistent with your eating schedule.

So, try to eat every day at the same time. In addition, try to keep your fasting schedule consistent every day.

This will make your intermittent fasting lifestyle easier to maintain and you will definitely lose weight as a result of following a consistent schedule.

If you find yourself without the time required to eat a proper meal to break your normal fast, make sure you at least eat something to keep your body on the fasting and eating cycle.

If you are exercising as well as doing intermittently fasting at the same time, it is important to make sure that you are eating more carbohydrates than healthy fats on the days you are working out.

However, on the days that you don't exercise simply eat more healthy fats than carbohydrates.

Simply, carbohydrates will give you the required energy you need to exercise as well as to recover from tough exercise workouts.

Also, it is important to make sure that every day you keep your protein intake at a steady level.

Protein is very important for growing and maintaining lean muscle so you don't want to lose muscle while fasting.

As a result, eat enough protein every day to feed your muscles.

It is important to mention that along your intermittent fasting journey, you need to make every attempt to stay away from processed foods whenever possible.

Processed foods are simply unhealthy for you even the so called "healthy" processed foods.

You instead want to focus on eating natural foods like fruits, vegetables and lean meats and include some healthy fats from avocados, eggs and walnuts.

One of the biggest benefits of the **16 Hours Fast: 8 Hours Eating Window** intermittent fasting approach is that it's extremely flexible so that it will work for a wide variety of schedules.

Most people find it helpful to either eat two large meals during the 8-hour feeding period or simply eat three smaller meals as that is the way most people are already programmed to eat.

Remember that on the days you are exercising as well as fasting, it is important to try and always break your fast with a mix of healthy protein, vegetables, and fruit.

If you generally go to the gym directly after you have broken your fast, it is important to include enough carbohydrates to give your muscles the energy they need to get the most out of your workouts.

If you are planning to exercise in the afternoon, it is usually best to break your fast a little before noontime and eat a healthy medium size meal.

After you finish eating wait about an hour or two before you exercise.

Then, after you exercise you can eat a larger meal to get all the necessary nutrients your body needs.

Remember to eat a good amount of complex carbohydrates after your workout so that your body is able to get the proper nutrition it needs as well as for recovery purposes.

You can even have a little dessert as long as it is in moderation.

Remember, fasting is different than dieting so you can still eat some of your favorite unhealthy foods but in moderation.

On days you do not plan on exercising, it is important to adjust your caloric intake appropriately.

So, on the days you don't exercise, simply reduce the amount of carbohydrates that you eat.

In addition, focus on eating lots of protein, dark green, leafy vegetables as well as some fruit in moderation.

Unlike on days you are exercising, the first meal you eat on rest days should be your largest meal of the day counting for about 40 percent of your daily calories.

Remember, because you are breaking your fast, you should be taking in more protein than any other food.

For your final meal during rest days, it is important to include a protein source that will take lots of time to digest which in turn means it will keep you full while you are fasting until the following morning/afternoon.

Some examples of good slow digesting protein foods are steak, beef, chicken and lamb.

It is important to state that eating good quality sources of protein like steak and beef provides the body with enough stored amino acids which prevents the body from breaking down muscle while you are fasting.

Eat-Stop-Eat (Another Intermittent Fasting Method)

This form of fasting can be considered the most beneficial to those who are already eating healthy but want to give their weight loss an extra boost.

On this type of Eat-Stop-Eat method, you don't eat anything for one or two days a week. This means that you do a full 24-hour fast once or twice a week.

During this period, you should only consume foods that have zero calories including black coffee, water and sugar-free gum.

When you are finished fasting, it is important not to eat too much food after you break your fast.

So, you want to break your 24-hour fast with a light meal and you want to avoid any binge eating as extended periods of fasting followed by binge eating can cause serious damage to your body.

As always, it is important to practice moderation and self-control to get the most out of the intermittent fasting.

Keep this in mind, to lose a pound of weight per week, all you need to do is burn 3,500 calories from exercise or reduce your calorie intake by 3,500 calories per week.

So, you can simply reduce your daily calorie intake by eating 500 less calories a day by fasting every day.

However, you can greatly decrease the number of calories you eat in a week by simply doing a 24 hour fast once or twice a week.

Going a full day without eating can be difficult for some people at first, but it is perfectly acceptable to work up to a full day of fasting by holding out as long as possible and increasing that amount of time with practice.

Some strategies for doing a 24-hour fast are:

- Drink a lot of water throughout a 24-hour fast.

- Stay busy and do something and don't just sit around or you will think about food.

- Try to sleep more. So, try to wake up later than usual and try to go to sleep earlier than usual.

- Try to do 24-hour fast when there are no social events or important holidays going on.

When first starting this Eat-Stop-Eat approach to intermittent fasting you may experience fatigue, headaches or feelings of anger or anxiousness.

Simply fatigue, headaches, or feelings of anger or anxiousness are all common side-effects of doing a 24-hour fast.

If for some reason you think you need to break your 24-hour fast then simply do so and try another 24-hour fast a few days later.

It is important to state that as you continue to practice more and more 24-hour fasts, any negative side-effects you may have experienced will diminish as your body adjusts to this intermittent fasting approach.

Keep in mind that after completing a full 24-hour fast, it will be natural to have the desire to go and binge on all kinds of foods for your fist meal.

Well you must have the self-control to fight these urges since not only is binge eating bad for you but binge eating can easily undo all your hard work from the previous 24-hour fast you just completed.

So, practice self-discipline and make your fasting worth the effort.

The Warrior Diet (Intermittent Fasting Method)

The Warrior Diet uses the **16 hours of fasting and 8-hour eating window** intermittent fasting approach.

Remember, the **16 hours of fasting and 8-hour eating window** intermittent fasting approach consists of 16 hours of fasting followed by an 8-hour eating period.

However, the Warrior Diet kicks it up a notch by recommending that you fast for roughly 20 hours every day followed by a 4-hour eating window.

So, on the Warrior Diet you will fast for 20 hours then you will try to get all of your calories from one meal during the 4-hour eating window.

This form of intermittent fasting approach follows the belief that humans are naturally nocturnal eaters.

Therefore, eating at night helps the body more easily process the nutrients it needs.

So, for example, you will fast from 8:00 PM - 4:00 PM the following day.

Then you will have a 4-hour eating window between 4:00 PM – 8:00 PM.

In this case, fasting is a bit of a misnomer as during the 20-hour period you are allowed to eat a serving of raw vegetables or fruits and maybe a serving of protein if you just can't otherwise endure the entire 20-hour fast.

However, you will be breaking your fast so you will not get the same benefits as if you would have successfully completed the 20-hour fast without eating any food.

One benefit of this long 20-hour Warrior Diet fast is that it simply works because it causes the body's natural nervous system to activate a "flight" or "fight" response which in turn increases your natural levels of alertness and increases energy while at the same time increasing the amount of fat you burn.

The one large meal that you have in the evening during your 4-hour eating window allows your body to focus on repairing itself and helps your muscles recover from any strenuous exercise workouts.

When following the Warrior Diet, it is important to start each evening meal with vegetables, followed by protein, healthy fats and carbohydrates.

So, you want to break your 20-hour fast by slowly eating light foods like vegetables followed by some proteins then fats and carbohydrates.

The Warrior Diet is popular for two reasons:

I.   First, the fact that a few small and reasonable snacks are allowed during the fasting process making this type of fasting attractive to those who are attempting this fasting approach for the first time.

II.   Second, nearly everyone who attempts this form of fasting reports a significant amount of increased energy throughout the day as well as an increase in the amount of fat lost per week.

On the other hand, the relatively long 20-hour fast can make it difficult for some people to go for long periods of time without eating.

It is important to state that the timing of the large meal during the 4-hour eating window can also make it difficult for some people to follow because it can naturally interfere with some social engagements.

So, if a person does a 20-hour fast from 8:00 PM until 4:00 PM the following day that means the person only has a very small 4-hour eating window to eat from.

So, a person that has a social life and likes to go out late in the evening may find it hard to follow a 20-hour fast.

However, because intermittent fasting is so flexible a person can decide to do a shorter fast like a 16 hour fast instead of a 20 hour fast.

The various intermittent fasting types and schedules are endless so even if a person lives a very social life that person can still live a fasting lifestyle.

The best thing that you can do is to simply try the Warrior Diet and see if it is suitable for you.

If you try the Warrior Diet and you determine that it is not for you, then you have other intermittent fasting options that you can choose from.

Fat Loss Forever (Intermittent Fasting Method)

The Fat Loss Forever form of intermittent fasting combines other types of fasting for the purpose of creating something rather unique.

The good news is that you get a cheat day every week.

The bad news is that it is followed by a 36-hour fast with the remainder of the week being split between a (**16 hours of fasting and 8-hour eating window**) fasting schedule and a (**20 Hours of fasting and 4-hour eating window**) fasting schedule.

For this intermittent fasting variation, it is important to schedule your exercise rest days during the 36-hour fast because if you attempt to exercises during your 36-hour fast you can easily get hungry and anxious from not eating as well as headaches and even some mood swings.

In addition, it is important that you stay extremely busy during your 36-hour fast in order to help combat your hunger.

If you find it hard to control your appetite on cheat days, then this form of intermittent fasting may not be for you since it requires you to go from eating anything you want on a cheat day to then fasting for 36-hours straight.

In the beginning, it is important not to try and last the entire 36 hours without eating any food.

Instead, you will need to slowly build up your body's tolerance for fasting for 36 hours straight.

As such, it is usually better to start with another form of intermittent fasting and work up to the **Fat Loss Forever Method** after your body has become used to fasting for 16 hours or more.

Remember to always fast responsibly and never push your body to the point where you feel physically ill.

Also, remember that it is important to fast on a specific set schedule every day so that your body can slowly adjust to your fasting lifestyle.

Alternate Day Diet (Intermittent Fasting Method)

This form of intermittent fasting actually means you never have to go long without food. Basically, every other day you don't fast and instead you eat your meals at no specific time.

However, on your fasting days you can only eat one-fifth of the calories you consume on your non-fasting days.

For example, the average daily caloric consumption is between 2,000 and 2,500 calories which means you will only be able to eat between 400 and 500 calories on your fasting days.

Now if you enjoy exercising every day, then this form of intermittent fasting may not be for you since you will have to severely limit your workouts on the days you fast as a result of the very few calories you will be consuming.

It is important to state that when you first start this form of intermittent fasting, the easiest way to make it through the low-calorie days is by simply eating a good source of protein, complex carbohydrates and some vegetables.

You also want to make sure to drink a lot of water since water will keep you feeling full. In addition, stay busy and try to sleep more.

Consider even taking an afternoon nap if possible to avoid from getting hungry.

What many people discover by using this form of intermittent fasting is that they will quickly lose a lot of weight.

However, you want to keep in mind that you want to slowly ease into intermittent fasting because you don't want to shock your body too much too soon.

In addition, you don't want to lose any lean muscle mass by losing too much weight too fast.

If you do attempt the **Alternate Day Fasting Method**, it is extremely important to eat wholesome healthy meals on the days you don't fast so that your body gets all the required nutrients it needs.

Keep in mind that binge eating will not only negate any progress you have made, but it can also cause serious damage to your body if continued over time.

Irregularly Skipping Meals (Intermittent Fasting Method)

If you are interested in trying out the benefits of intermittent fasting for yourself, but you have an irregular schedule or are not sure if it is for you, then skipping a meal or two now and then may be the best type of intermittent fasting for you.

As previously discussed, getting into a fasting routine is important to see the maximum results for your effort, but that doesn't mean that fasting occasionally doesn't come with some benefits as well.

What's more, once you have tried skipping a meal now and then you will see for yourself just how easy fasting can be.

In addition, skipping a meal now and then and slowly easing into intermittent fasting will lead to more positive changes with your health down the line.

As you can see there are so many intermittent fasting options available that you can choose from.

Simply find an intermittent fasting approach that fits your schedule and give fasting a try.

If you stay consistent with your intermittent fasting schedule you are most certainly going to achieve your weight loss goals.

Chapter 3: Intermittent Fasting Health Benefits

Other than weight loss, you can receive other benefits from intermittent fasting in many other ways.

For example, researchers have concluded that intermittent fasting will help you live a longer life as a result of practicing intermittent fasting.

What intermittent fasting does is that the more you practice intermittent fasting and the longer you fast for, the more you divert energy away from being used to break down unnecessary food or foods you constantly eat.

In addition, intermittent fasting improves your biological functions.

For example, you will be more alert, more aware and have more energy as a result of practicing intermittent fasting.

Intermittent fasting will also naturally develop human growth hormone (HGH).

Human growth hormone is a hormone that is similar to steroids but the difference is that human growth hormone is naturally developed by the body instead of having steroids injected to the body.

What this means is that you will feel younger, you will not get tired very easily and you will be able to recover from strenuous workouts faster as a result of naturally developing human growth hormone from intermittent fasting.

Basically, human growth hormone is the "Fountain of Youth" and many athletes, movie stars and wealthy people inject themselves with expensive human growth hormone injections so that they can feel rejuvenated.

Just remember, that when you do plan to begin practicing intermittent fasting that you don't in any way let yourself starve or get to hungry.

As you begin to fast, the body will send emergency signals to your brain telling it that it needs food.

However, these emergency signals will slowly diminish once your body adjusts to its intermittent fasting routine.

Here are some other benefits regarding intermittent fasting:

- *Improved Brain Health:* Your brain hormone—BDNF—also known as brain-derived "neurotropic" factor—is a protein that can aid in the growth of new nerve cells.

  So, as you practice intermittent fasting, you also grow more new nerve cells in your brain which can provide protection against Alzheimer's and Parkinson's disease.

- *Cancer:* Studies using animals have suggested intermittent fasting can be beneficial in the prevention of cancer.

- *Healthy Heart:* Your blood triglycerides, LDL cholesterol, insulin resistance, and blood sugar each present a huge risk for heart ailments or disease.

  However, all of these issues with your heart can be greatly reduced as a result of practicing intermittent fasting.

- *Inflammation:* Chronic diseases are driven by inflammation. However, research studies have shown that intermittent fasting helps to reduce inflammation in the body.

So, your body will be capable of repairing and healing itself as well as recovering more quickly if you practice some form of intermittent fasting.

- *Insulin Resistance:* Both your blood sugar levels and your insulin levels can be greatly reduced by simply practicing intermittent fasting.

  Simply, intermittent fasting protects you against type 2 diabetes.

- *Anti-Aging:* Researchers tested animals such as rats to see what benefits they would receive by placing them on an intermittent fasting diet.

  What researches determined was that the rats that were placed on an intermittent fasting diet lived 36% to 83% longer than rats that were not placed on an intermittent fasting diet.

- *Lower Stress Levels:* Cortisol is a hormone your body produces when you are stressed. However, your cortisol levels are greatly reduced as a result of practicing intermittent fasting.

- *Fatty Acid Oxidation:* The more you eat the more energy you eat. As a result, your body will burn the food you eat as energy instead of the stored fats in your body.

  However, when a person practices intermittent fasting, the body will burn stored fats in the body as energy as a result of the body having less food to burn as energy.

So, when the body burns stored fat as energy, weight loss occurs.

Note: These are some benefits of intermittent fasting resulting from studies that have been done on this fascinating lifestyle.

However, more research needs to be provided using more human testing during the fasting process.

Chapter 4: The Process

While intermittent fasting is undeniably beneficial, it can be difficult to get started or to see through to the point where your body adapts to a new eating schedule.

The following tips and tricks can help set you on the path to success with intermittent fasting:

- **Have a conversation with yourself:** Intermittent fasting has a wide variety of proven benefits, but it is not for everyone.

  Before you attempt to fast, it is important to have a real dialogue with yourself.

  Consider your level of self-discipline and your current attachment to food.

  Also consider any regular activities that would make fasting difficult for you, your general lifestyle, and your level of exercise.

  So simply make a decision to try intermittent fasting and stick to with it.

  In the beginning it will be hard but eventually it will become easier so decide to make a commitment and practice intermittent fasting.

- **Watch your response:** While it is important to be aware of how your body is responding during intermittent fasting, it is very important to aware of the beginning phase of intermittent fasting.

The initial phase of intermittent fasting will be tough but simply monitor how your body is adjusting to its new eating schedule as well as how you feel during the initial phase.

Some discomfort is to be expected for the first three to four weeks, but anything longer or more severe should be discussed with a doctor as soon as possible.

- **The early days will have ups and downs:** While your body adjusts to intermittent fasting, there will be times where you are losing weight and times where your body is trying to hold on to every calorie it has.

  This is natural and to be expected as your body realigns its hormone levels.

- **Drink lots of water:** Not only will water help you feel full throughout your fast, staying hydrated is beneficial for staying healthy.

  Try to drink at least one gallon of water per day.

- **Caffeine naturally suppresses your appetite:** Research has shown that black coffee suppresses a person's appetite and does not interfere with intermittent fasting.

  However, the same cannot be said for most 0-calorie caffeinated beverages.

  In addition, artificial sweeteners have been shown to cause some health problems.

- **Keep yourself busy:** Plain and simple, stay busy while fasting! Make sure that the latter parts of your fast aren't just spent waiting around to eat.

Intermittent fasting has the possibility to be either extremely difficult or surprisingly easy depending solely on how much of the time you spend thinking about food.

What is more important is that you find ways to occupy your mind and stay busy in order to prevent sitting around thinking about when you are going to eat.

- **Start each fast off right:** Once you finish eating you are done eating and that's it!

  You brush your teeth and you simply stay busy and keep your mind off of food.

  One thing that you can do to keep yourself occupied is schedule your chores, your daily work and routines around your fasting schedule.

  You will eventually develop a positive habit of knowing when you are going to eat and when it is time to focus on your daily activities.

- **Make it work for you:** Intermittent fasting can work around any type of schedule which is what makes it so great.

  If you don't like eating too late in the afternoon or you don't like eating dinner too early, simply experiment with different fasting schedules until you find a routine that works for you.

  Intermittent fasting should be about losing weight in a slow, healthy and suitable manner.

- **Don't expect results overnight:** As previously discussed, it will take some time for your body to fully adjust to your new fasting schedule.

In addition, it will take a few weeks to see some results from intermittent fasting.

However, be consistent with your fasting schedule as well as patient and you are bound to see some great results from intermittent fasting.

Keep this in mind, try intermittent fasting consistently for at least one month before rendering judgment on this healthy lifestyle.

- **Vary your schedule (if needed):** After you have given your body time to adjust to an intermittent fasting schedule, determine whether your fasting schedule is suitable for you.

  If you have determined that you are not happy with your fasting schedule, simply adjust your fasting schedule and experiment with other fasting schedules until you find a schedule that works best for you.

- **Start slow:** If you find that you are having difficulty starting a very discipline intermittent fasting routine, simply try delay eating your breakfast every week by one hour.

  For example, this week you will eat breakfast at 7:00 AM.

  Then next week, you will eat breakfast at 8:00 AM.

  Then the following week you will eat breakfast at 9:00 AM.

  Eventually, you will all together skip breakfast and simply build up your fasting tolerance to wait until 12:00 PM to eat lunch.

  This is how you slowly ease into intermittent fasting.

In addition, I honestly think that this is the best and easiest method for getting started with intermittent fasting.

- **Keep intermittent fasting to yourself:** While there is plenty of scientific evidence that supports the benefits of intermittent fasting, there are still plenty of skeptics out there.

  Skeptics and negative people are something that you don't need, especially when you are first going to begin your intermittent fasting journey.

  First simply focus on developing a fasting schedule that is suitable for you.

  Then later as you start to see results from you fasting lifestyle, you can slowly share your knowledge about intermittent fasting.

  There will always be nonbelievers when it comes to intermittent fasting.

  But remember, you don't have to explain yourself to anyone about your fasting lifestyle.

  Instead, silently succeed at achieving your weight loss goals and maybe show a before and after picture to any skeptics you may encounter.

- **Start the day by drinking water:** Whenever your body sends signs that you are hungry your body is actually telling you that it is thirsty.

  If you ignore any signs from your body telling you that it is thirsty your body will eventually send signs that it is hungry when it actually isn't.

So, what you have to do while you are fasting is to simply drink a lot of water throughout the day and limit your intake of water in the early evening or a few hours before you go to sleep.

Keep this in mind…the more water you drink throughout the day the less hungry you will feel throughout the day.

So, start the morning off by drinking at least a half of liter of water as soon as you wake up.

Drinking this amount of water is an excellent way to quench your body's thirst from the past seven or eight hours that you have been asleep.

In addition, immediately drinking water as soon as you wake up in the morning gets the body to restart and ready for the day ahead.

- **Don't take on too much, too fast:** Even if you think you feel fine when you first begin an intermittent fast routine, it is important to always give your body the necessary time it needs to adjust and recover.

In the beginning never go more than two days straight without eating.

You want to slowly let your body adjust to fasting for 12, 14 and eventually 16 hours or more.

Keep in mind that intermittent fasting is about giving your body a break from eating and it is not about starving yourself.

- **Splurge when you want:** Remember that you need to burn 3,500 calories to lose one pound of fat per week, but how you do that is up to you.

  So, keep in mind that if you want to have a delicious dessert or an unhealthy cheat meal throughout the week, that is perfectly fine.

  Just make sure that you make an effort to continue fasting throughout the week in order to continue with your fat loss progress.

- **Distract yourself:** Distracting yourself and keeping busy is especially important in the beginning phase of starting an intermittent fasting routine.

  Simply your body will begin the process of adapting to your new eating habits and so you have to make sure that you don't just sit around thinking about what time you are going to eat or what food you are going to eat.

  It is better to be productive while fasting because it is at this very moment that you have the most energy and are most alert as a result of fasting.

  So, work on an important project or complete a difficult work assignment while fasting because this is the moment when your mind is most focused.

- **Add protein to your meals:** Eating good quality protein while fasting is very important.

  What protein does is that it helps you to stay full for longer periods of time.

In addition, protein will feed your muscles with the nutrients they need in order for them to stay strong and lean.

Good quality protein from steak, beef and chicken will take quite a few hours for your body to digest.

Therefore, make sure to include good quality protein in all of your meals while fasting.

If you find yourself unable to go through 10 hours without eating, then it might be a sign that you should add more protein to your diet.

- **Try Branched Chain Amino Acids (BCAA's):** For those individuals that strength train while intermittent fasting, studies show that a Branched Chain Amino Acids (BCAA's) supplement will stimulate additional fat loss while at the same time preventing lean muscle from being consumed as the body tries to feed itself.

  It is important to state that Branched Chain Amino Acids (BCAA's) are recommend for people that exercise especially for people that do a lot of strength training exercises.

  Otherwise, Branched Chain Amino Acids (BCAA's) are not needed nor required for your average person that simply practices intermittent fasting.

- **Intermittent fasting is not an excuse to eat poorly:** Intermittent fasting works on the principle that eating fewer calories than you burn is a great way to lose weight.

  However, this theory falls apart if you use the fact that you are fasting as an excuse to eat nothing but junk food when you are eating.

Self-control and self-discipline are both equally important when it comes to eating properly while practicing intermittent fasting.

Intermittent fasting has so many health benefits so there is no point for eating unhealthy food while fasting.

Now it is ok to have a cheat meal or some dessert every now and then but to simply fast for the sake of eating unhealthy food does not make any sense.

If you are serious about getting lean and fit with intermittent fasting then it is best to be disciplined with your fasting schedule and your eating habits.

Otherwise, what is the point of fasting?

- **Break your fast the right way:** The quality of the food you eat after you break your fast is important for ensuring that you are feeding your body the necessary nutrients that it needs.

  In addition, eating good quality healthy food will even accelerate your weight loss because you will be consuming foods that are low in fat unlike unhealthy foods which are full of sugar and fat.

  You will be surprised how easy it is to lose weight with intermittent fasting especially when you consume the right healthy foods and you remain consistent with your healthy intermittent fasting lifestyle.

- **Consider the difference between "head hunger" and "body hunger:"** As you get used to the process of intermittent fasting, you will become acquainted with two types of hunger.

The first type of hunger is "head hunger" which means that your mind is simply telling you that you are hungry because you are bored or because you are thirsty or because you smell food.

The second kind of hunger is "body hunger" which means that your body specifically your stomach is growling and telling you that you are hungry.

It is important to know when you are truly hungry and when you "think" you are hungry.

It is also important to state that even though your stomach may be growling trying to tell you that you are hungry, you can still go a few more hours without eating.

So, don't be afraid to let yourself get a little hungry.

The problem with most people is that they believe that if they don't eat food every 3 or 4 hours they are going to starve or faint and this is simply not true.

- **Learn what your body is saying:** Be aware of your cravings.

More importantly be aware of your cravings that make you think you are hungry.

While everybody has a craving for some type of food, it is important to understand that although you may crave a certain food, that does not mean that you are hungry.

In addition, if you do crave a certain type of food then you can simply eat a small portion of it but only as part of your eating window.

So, don't break your fasting routine for the sake of giving in to a food craving.

Instead, make every effort to control your cravings of certain foods and don't let food control your eating habits.

Remember, true weight loss and the practice of intermittent fasting require discipline and commitment and if you don't develop discipline with your eating habits and make a commitment to lose weight, then you will simply never achieve your health and fitness goals.

- **Exercise in moderation:** Dieting works by taking in fewer calories than you burn, each and every day.

As such, if you are trying one of the intermittent fasting approaches that involves fasting for 24-hours or more, then it is extremely important to adjust your exercise workouts around your fasting schedule.

For example, you can have two good nutritious meals on the days you exercise and on the days you don't exercise, you can do a full 24-hour fast or simply have one big meal.

Remember that when you exercise, your body requires fuel. So, on the days you exercise, you need to make sure you feed your body adequate protein and carbs as well as healthy fats and vegetables.

If you don't feed your body the necessary foods it needs when you exercise, then your body will use your muscles as fuel resulting in muscle loss.

- **Respect intermittent fasting:** Those individuals who have suffered from eating disorders or who may have an eating disorder should stay away from intermittent fasting as it can easily lead to more serious issues.

  For example, people who suffer from binge eating and purging, which are signs of bulimia, may believe that binge eating and purging is a form of intermittent fasting when it is not.

  In addition, some individuals may thing it is ok to binge eat after fasting for 16 hours when in reality it is not.

  Instead, intermittent fasting is a safe and healthy lifestyle that has many health benefits that can be practiced by many people.

  However, it is important to never abuse intermittent fasting and to always be aware of any eating disorders such as binge eating and purging.

Chapter 5: Weight Loss and Intermittent Fasting

When it comes to weight loss it is important to know how many calories your body needs each and every day.

In addition, you also need to adopt a realistic approach to weight loss in order to achieve your weight loss goals.

One way to keep track of your weight loss goals is by using a Body Mass Index (BMI) calculator.

A Body Mass Index (BMI) calculator will tell you how much fat you have on your body.

You can simply go online and type Body Mass Index and you will then see a calculator.

You simply enter your sex, height, weight and age on the calculator and you will immediately get your results regarding how much body fat you have on your body.

In addition, the Body Mass Index calculator will tell you if you are underweight, normal weight, overweight or obese.

Some Body Mass Index calculators may even ask you how much daily exercise you are getting.

In addition, some Body Mass Index calculators may even tell you how many calories you need to eat every day in order to lose weight or maintain your weight.

Another tool to use for helping you keep track of your fat loss goals while practicing intermittent fasting is a Calorie Calculator.

A Calorie Calculator will help you determine how many calories you need to eat each and every day.

You can simply go online and type Calorie Calculator and you will be able to choose from a list of calculators.

Because most food products you purchase will have ingredient panels listing the number of calories the food has per serving, it will be easy for you to use a Calorie Counter for keeping track of how many calories you eat each and every day.

Using both a Body Mass Index calculator as well as a Calorie Counter are two great tools to use as part of your intermittent fasting plan.

Maintain a Healthy Diet Plan

Making intermittent fasting a part of your life is an excellent way to lose weight.

However, eating healthy food while practicing intermittent fasting is very important for achieving the best weight loss results.

Below is a list of some healthy foods you should consume as part of your intermittent fasting eating plan:

- Whole Fruits like blueberries and apples.

- Healthy Fats like Avocados and Olive Oil

- Protein foods such as eggs, poultry, lean meats, seafood, nuts and soy products

- A variety of vegetables like spinach, kale, sweet potatoes, lettuce, broccoli, etc.,

It is important to state that you want to eat whole, natural foods and stay away from processed and prepacked foods because these types of foods contain a lot of salt, sugar and other unhealthy ingredients.

Here are some recommendations that may help you with your weight loss goals:

- Consume less than 10% of your daily calories from saturated fats. Some foods with saturated fats are butter, processed meats and hydrogenated oils.

- Eat less than 10% of your daily intake of calories from added sugars.

- Limit your sodium consumption. Sodium consumption should be less than 2,300 mg (milligrams) per day.

- Try to eliminate or reduce your drinking of alcohol. Alcohol, especially beer has a lot of empty calories.

What Not to Eat

With all the talk on the importance of natural foods, you may be wondering what foods should be avoided to make intermittent fast more effective?

As a general rule, the following foods should be avoided or at least limited as much as possible:

- **Processed Meats**: While eating quality protein is an important part of a healthy diet, eating protein from processed meats is extremely unhealthy.

Processed meats tend to be lower in protein and have high amounts of sodium. Eating foods with lots of sodium can cause a variety of health risks including asthma and heart disease.

It is important to always choose lean cuts of quality protein over processed meats.

- **Non-organic potatoes:** While sweet potatoes are a good source of carbohydrates non-organic potatoes should not be eaten.

  Non-organic potatoes are treated with chemicals while they are still in the ground.

  Non-organic potatoes are treated again before they head to the store to ensure they stay "fresh" as long as possible.

  The chemicals that are sprayed on non-organic potatoes have been shown to increase the risk of health issues like autism, asthma, birth defects, learning disabilities, Parkinson's and Alzheimer's disease as well as multiple types of cancer.

- **Farm-raised salmon**: Much like processed meat, farm-raised salmon is not a healthy food choice.

  When salmon are raised in tubs of water near one another for a prolonged period of time, they lose much of their natural vitamin D while picking up traces of PCB (toxic chemical compounds), DDT, carcinogens, and bromine.

  Although more expensive but way healthier, choose wild caught fish if possible.

- **Non-organic milk:** Non-organic milk should be eliminated from your diet.

Despite being touted as part of a balanced diet, non-organic milk is routinely found to be full of growth hormones as well as puss as a result of the cows being over-milked.

The growth hormones leave behind antibiotics which can, in turn, make it more difficult for the human body to counter infections as well as causing an increased chance of colon cancer, prostate cancer, and breast cancer.

Try drinking some healthy milk such as organic milk or simply drink milk with no hormones.

Both organic milk and milk with no hormones will give you the necessary nutrients your body needs without consuming any unhealthy growth hormones.

- **White Flour:** White flour should be eliminated from your diet.

  Much like processed meats, by the time white flour is done being produced it is completely devoid of any nutritional value.

  When eaten as part of a regular diet, white flour has been shown to increase a woman's chance of breast cancer by a shocking 200 percent.

As you can see by the foods mentioned above, these are just a few of the reasons why processed foods should be eliminated from your intermittent fasting lifestyle.

Keep in mind that processed foods can be considered any food items which contain preservatives, chemical colors, flavorings, additives or chemicals which change its texture.

An additional extremely important warning sign of unhealthy food is when a food item contains a large amount of refined carbohydrates.

Some foods that contain a lot of refined carbohydrates are cookies, cakes, breads, pastries, ice-cream and more so start eliminating these foods from your diet!

The secret to losing weight and getting lean is to simply eat whole natural foods.

In addition, take the time to read the food labels and check the ingredients that are listed on food labels.

You can also begin to use what's called "portion control" for eliminating fat from your body and maintaining your levels of leanness.

"Portion control" is simply a method of measuring or weighting the amount of food you eat.

You can use a food scale to measure your food and keep track of how much food you are eating at every meal.

In addition, you can use small plates instead of big plates to eat your food.

Using small plates to eat your food will condition you to eat less food.

Keep this in mind along your fat loss journey…how bad do you want to lose weight?

Do you want to look like everyone else; fat, overweight, obese with several health issues?

Simply, decide to make a choice to lose weight in a safe controlled manner and stick to your decision.

So, make a commitment to a healthy lifestyle and if you have a cheat meal or two along your fat loss journey, well simply immediately resume your fasting lifestyle but stay focused on your weight loss goals.

Also, write down your health and fitness goals and read over them every day so that you can remain focused on achieving your weight loss goals.

Chapter 6: Intermittent Fasting and Nutrition

How to Boost Your Metabolism

For some people losing weight may be difficult. However, intermittent fasting is a great way to achieve your fat loss goals.

But, it is important to state you can lose weight even faster by eating specific foods while practicing intermittent fasting.

Below is a list of some foods that you should specifically eat in order to rapidly increase fat loss:

Protein-Rich Food Groups

Your body will need more energy to digest these protein-rich foods:

- Eggs
- Seeds and nuts – specifically walnuts and almonds
- Legumes – specifically chickpeas, lentils and kidney beans,
- Fish – specifically freshwater salmon and sardines
- Meat – specifically skinless chicken breast and chicken tenders as well as lean beef like top sirloin and beef tenderloins

It important to state that eating good quality protein will make you feel full much longer than other foods and possibly prevent you from overeating.

It is also important to state that eating these protein-rich roods will cause a thermal effect in your body.

A thermic effect of food is referred to as TEF which is the number of calories required by your body to absorb/digest nutrients received by your meals.

So, when you eat foods like chicken breast, beef and almonds your metabolism will work faster as a result of your body using energy to break down these foods.

In addition to eating protein-rich foods, eating two big healthy meals a day while practicing intermittent fasting will cause your body to use more energy to break down food.

So, while your body uses more energy to break down two big meals a day, your metabolism will be working faster which means you will also lose weight faster.

Essential Vitamins and Minerals

Vitamins such as zinc, iron, and selenium are essential for the human body to function properly.

Research shows that a diet low in zinc, iron, and selenium reduces the ability of the thyroid gland to produce crucial hormones.

If the ability of the thyroid gland to produce crucial hormones is affected then your body's metabolism will slow down.

However, if you want to make sure you get enough zinc, iron, and selenium it is best to eat seeds, nuts, legumes, meat, and seafood.

In addition, here are some other nutritious foods that you can eat to help boost your metabolism:

- **Chili Peppers:** There is a chemical found in chili peppers called capsaicin which helps boost the body's metabolism.

The capsaicin will increase the fat and calories you burn during your intermittent fasting plan.

Twenty research studies show that you would lose/burn approximately fifty extra calories a day by eating chili peppers or foods with capsaicin.

However, now all researchers agree with this theory.

What can be said about chili peppers is to simply add them to your intermittent fasting diet and see if they help with your weight loss goals.

- **Legumes:** This food group includes peanuts, lentils, chickpeas, beans, and peas which are extremely high in protein levels in comparison to other plant foods.

  According to research studies, eating high protein foods such as legumes will result in the human body burning a larger number of calories in order to digest them.

  This study was compared against participants that ate lower-protein foods.

  More recent studies have indicated that participants who consumed a legume-rich diet for eight weeks increased their body's metabolism and lost more than 1.5 times more weight versus another group of participants that didn't eat a legume-rich diet.

  So, what can be said about legumes is to simply try to make them part of your intermittent fasting diet plan.

- **Coffee:** If you drink coffee, the caffeine levels in the coffee can help increase the body's metabolic rate by approximately 11%.

Studies have shown that consumption of a minimum of 270 mg of caffeine, about three cups of coffee, will burn away an additional 100 calories daily.

So, drinking coffee can be good for you. In addition, drinking coffee will most definitely boost your metabolism and help you burn more calories.

However, make sure your coffee is sugar-free coffee while practicing intermittent fasting because sugar is bad for you and you want to eliminate as much sugar from your diet as possible.

- **Tea:** Tea is often recommended for its health benefits such as providing antioxidants, reducing heart attacks and strokes as well as helping protect the bones of the body.

  But in addition to these health benefits, tea is also known to help with weight loss.

  Some teas have less caffeine then coffee but at the same time these teas help speed up the body's metabolism which leads to weight loss.

  It is estimated that an additional 100 calories can be burned daily by drinking specifically green and oolong tea.

  Drinking these teas will speed up your metabolism by four to ten percent.

  Try to make drinking green and oolong tea as part of your fasting diet.

Not only with green and oolong tea provide your body with many health benefits but you will also lose some weight by drinking these two healthy teas.

Chapter 7: Intermittent Fasting Methods for Everyday Living

Method (16 hours of fasting and 8-hour eating window) or the Lean Gains Protocol

The **16 hours of fasting and 8-hour eating window** method or sometimes referred to as the Lean Gains protocol is all about having an eight-hour eating window and then fasting for the next 16 hours.

So basically, you can eat one, two or even three meals during an eight-hour eating period. But, once your eight-hour eating period ends, you then fast for 16 hours.

The **16 hours of fasting and 8-hour eating window** intermittent fasting method was made popular by famous movie star Hugh Jackman from the movie Wolverine.

Hugh Jackman made the headlines when he was interviewed about his diet for his action movies.

Hugh Jackman stated that he practiced the **16 hours of fasting and 8-hour eating window** intermittent fasting method as a way to lean down for his movie roles.

What has become interesting in the past few years is that the **16 hours of fasting and 8-hour eating window** intermittent fasting method has become the most preferred method for weight loss when it comes to fasting.

The **16 hours of fasting and 8-hour eating window** intermittent fasting method is very easy for most people to follow because most people will be sleeping for approximately eight of those fasting hours.

In addition, most people start their fast two or three hours before they go to sleep.

Many people have also stated that they are not hungry immediately upon waking up so they can easily postpone eating until lunchtime.

To practice the 16:8 intermittent fasting method you must keep in mind that your meals should be slightly larger than normal and your meals should consist of healthy food choices.

Another important point to mention is that while fasting on the **16 hours of fasting and 8-hour eating window** method, there must be absolutely zero consumption of food while fasting because consuming any calories even small amounts will interrupt the fasting process.

It is important to state that if you are overweight and live a sedentary lifestyle you should avoid most starchy carbohydrates like bread and pasta.

In addition, you must keep in mind that you only have an eight-hour eating window so you have to make sure to eat all of your calories during this time period to ensure the success with the 16:8 fasting method.

Many individuals on the **16 hours of fasting and 8-hour eating window** method can fit two large meals into the eight-hour eating window.

But it is important to remember that daily consistency of practicing the 16:8 method is what is most important for achieving success with this intermittent fasting method.

A study performed by the Obesity Society concluded that if you fast then eat your first meal around noontime your hunger yearnings will be greatly reduced for the remainder of the day.

At the same time, your body's fat-burning reserves will be used as energy as a result of fasting.

No matter what you may have heard about the **16 hours of fasting and 8-hour eating window** fasting method, you will not be as hungry once you have your fasting schedule as well as your meals properly planned for each and every day.

In addition, keep in mind that the real secret to the **16 hours of fasting and 8-hour eating window** method is daily consistency with your fasting schedule.

If you remain consistent with your fasting schedule you will most certainly achieve your weight loss goals.

You can use these sample meal plans as a guide for your fasting schedule:

Day 1
- **Morning:** Tea, water, or no sugar coffee is allowed.
- **Lunch:** Chicken Breast with black bean sauce, green veggies, and fruit.
- **Dinner:** Salmon and baked veggies with sweet potatoes. (If this is too much for one meal, simply eat half and save the rest for the following day.

Day 2: Repeat Day 1

Additional Tips
- **Sugar Substitutes:** Xylitol can replace sugar. Replace the coffee with black or green tea.

- **Stay Hydrated:** Drink plenty of tea, water, or coffee during the morning hours. It also helps prevent any hunger pains you may feel as a result of fasting. If possible, replace the coffee with black or green tea.

- **Sleep:** You need to have a full eight hours of sleep. It is advisable to avoid your cell phone and laptop (blue light) for up to an hour before you are ready to retire for the evening.

The Consistent Path to Fat Loss

The goal is to set your daily eating schedule to the same time every day.

By setting your daily eating schedule to the same time every day you program your body to adjust to a consistent eating schedule which prevents you from getting hungry.

If you often vary your eating schedule while practicing intermittent fasting, your hormones will be all over the place, resulting in your body holding onto unwanted weight.

It is also important to keep your protein levels consistent throughout your everyday fasting schedule.

In addition, it is a good idea to slightly increase your protein intake on days you do strenuous workouts such as strength training, swimming sprints or participating in CrossFit activities.

It is recommended that women should try to consume at least 55 grams of protein every day and men should try to consume at least 60 grams of protein per day.

If you consume the correct levels of protein and exercise regularly while taking in a steady amount of carbs, you should have all the energy needed on a daily basis.

However, if you are less inclined to exercise you should focus on eating healthy fats and minimize the number of carbs you eat.

When it comes to eating healthy fats such as avocados and walnuts, aim to eat approximately 0.7 grams of healthy fats for each pound of body weight.

In addition, it is best to avoid processed foods and unhealthy fats while choosing healthier, natural alternatives when possible.

If you are not an avid exerciser, then simply stick to your fasting schedule and your set meal plans and make sure not to accidentally overeat.

Eat-Stop-Eat (Fasting Method)

The Eat-Stop-Eat fasting method is all about fasting for 24 hours once or twice a week.

As an example, you would eat lunch on Wednesday around 12:00 PM and then you will fast until the following day, Thursday at 12:00 PM.

Once it is 12:00 PM on Thursday, you would then break your fast, each lunch and then have dinner around 6:30 PM.

So, after you complete a full 24-hour fast, you can then break your fast by following the 16:8 intermittent fasting method.

A lot of health professionals say that if you are able to fast for twenty hours, then that is sufficient to call it a full day of fasting.

However, if you can complete a full 24-hour fast then that is even better.

Now if you plan to do two 24-hour fasts in one week, you need to condition your body to adjust its calorie intake throughout the week.

For example, you can do one 24-hour fast on Monday then do another 24-hour fast on Friday.

This method of doing a 24-hour fast early in the week and then another 24-hour fast later in the week, allows your body time to receive a good amount of calories in-between 2 full 24-hour fasts.

One thing to keep in mind is that on the days that you are not doing a full 24-hour fast, you can simply follow the **16 hours of fasting and 8-hour eating window** intermittent fasting method so that you can make sure you consume a good amount of calories by eating at least two large meals during your eight-hour eating window.

Non-Fasting and Fasting Day Nutrients

Intermittent fasting can be practiced every day, seven days a week, 365 days a year.

Now how you adjust your intermittent fasting schedule is up to you. But many people have had much success with using the **16 hours of fasting and 8-hour eating window** method.

In addition, it is very possible to practice intermitting fasting every day using the **16 hours of fasting and 8-hour eating window** fasting method.

Keep in mind that if you choose not to fast on certain days of the week, simply try to control your food portions in order to prevent yourself from overeating.

In addition, on your non-fasting days, try to eat as healthy as possible making sure to eat leans cuts of quality protein as well as some healthy fats like avocados and a lot of vegetables.

On your fasting days, try to follow the **16 hours of fasting and 8-hour eating window** fasting method and limit yourself to 2 large healthy meals.

On your fasting days, make sure to drink a lot of water especially in the morning as soon as you wake up.

Drinking lots of water while you fast will keep you from feeling full preventing you from feeling hungry.

If you decide to exercise on the days you fast, simply try to eat healthy complex carbohydrates such as sweet potatoes or steel cut oats in order to make sure you have the necessary energy to get a good workout as well as to make sure you get the necessary nutrients you need to recover from a tough workout.

If you feel that you are struggling to lose weight while fasting, simply try to eliminate some foods from your diet like fruits and some carbohydrates and instead replace these foods with more protein, healthy fats and vegetables.

You can also use a food scale to weigh your food.

Actually, using a food scale to weight your food is one of the best ways to practice portion control.

Fluid Intake

Drinking enough water while practicing intermittent fasting is very important.

You can drink some sugar free coffee and tea but try to only drink water while fasting.

In addition, eliminate any fruit drinks, shakes, smoothies, fruit juices, and milk because these beverages are full of sugar and will increase your weight instead of helping you to lose weight.

It is also important to mention that if you condition yourself to only drink water every day, you will eliminate your craving for sugary drinks.

What many people don't seem to realize is that obesity and severe weight gain is a result of consuming too much sugar.

For example, the average American consumes too much sugar in their diet whether it is eating foods with lots of sugar or drinking beverages with lots of sugar.

So, remember to drink a lot of water both on you fasting days and your non-fasting days. In addition, eliminate sugary drinks from you fasting lifestyle.

Stay disciplined and focused with your intermittent fasting schedule and you will definitely achieve your weight loss goals.

Additional Tips

Intermittent fasting is one of the best ways to lose weight and keep it off.

As a result, here are some tips and strategies that may help you with your fasting lifestyle:

- Do not binge eat while practicing intermittent fasting. Binge eating will create havoc within your body so stay disciplined with your eating habits.

- Eliminate unhealthy processed foods from your diet and stick to whole, natural foods.

- Make exercise, specifically strength training exercises part of your fasting lifestyle. Intermittent fasting combined with strength training will truly get you lean and fit so go out and live a fasting fitness lifestyle.

- Eliminate unhealthy foods from your diet and focus on just eating a few handful of healthy foods that you truly enjoy eating often.

- Develop the habit of cooking for yourself. In addition, make cooking simple by preparing easy to make meals that you can prepare in an hour or less.

- Find like-minded people that are also on a journey to lose weight and look great. This can be a weight loss social group you meet with once a week or an online group that discusses weight loss strategies and tips.

- Eliminate people from your life that may try to sabotage your weight loss goals. This includes family members and friends.

- Stay consistent with your fasting schedule as well as your scheduled meals.

- In the beginning give yourself two weeks for your body and mind to get used to your new intermittent fasting schedule. After two weeks, slowly make any adjustments to your fasting schedule as needed.

- No matter what happens, don't quit intermittent fasting. Have a cheat meal now and then but then immediately go right back to following your fasting schedule.

The Warrior Diet (Intermittent Fasting Method)

It is believed that the name of this fasting method is a reflection of our ancient ancestors who were natural nocturnal eaters.

As a variation from the **16 hours of fasting and 8-hour eating window** method, the Warrior Diet is a fasting method that promotes eating one healthy meal a day.

In addition, this one meal a day is usually dinner.

The Warrior Diet works according to the human 24-hour rhythm also known as the circadian rhythm.

The circadian rhythm is simply the "body's clock" that works in a cycle telling us when to sleep, when to wake up and when to eat.

What is great about the Warrior Diet is that because only one large meal is eaten specifically at night, the body goes through a long fast which cleanses the body and removes any harmful toxins from the body.

Because only one large meal is eaten for dinner, a person will feel very alert during the day as well as have a lot of energy as a result of fasting throughout the night and day.

The Warrior Diet Daytime Feeding Schedule

For the Warrior Diet to be effective, you need to consume very little to no food during the day.

You can maybe eat a small piece of fruit or a handful of walnuts but that is it.

Many people may say that eating a small piece of fruit or a handful of walnuts is breaking the fast and that is true.

However, this is what our ancient ancestors used to do.

Our ancient ancestors used to eat one large meal for dinner and during the day they would sometimes eat a small piece of fruit or some nuts.

It is highly recommended that for the Warrior Diet to truly be effective it is better to eliminate ALL food during the day and simply stick to eating one large meal at night.

In addition, it is very important to drink lots and lots of water throughout the day in order to remain hydrated as well as to help you stay full.

Nighttime Feeding Frenzy

Back when our ancient ancestors used to practice the Warrior Diet, they would eat dinner like kings and sleep like babies at night.

As a result, the Warrior Diet requires you to eat a very large but nutritious meal at night.

You can eat as much food as you like but make sure your large meal is balanced with lean cuts of quality protein, healthy fats as well as complex carbohydrates and vegetables.

It is important to eliminate all processed foods as well as sugar from the Warrior Diet.

In addition, when you feel full or have satisfied your hunger or if you become more thirsty than hungry it is time to stop eating.

Follow the Warrior Diet Rules

Start your meal with a salad, lean cuts of protein, and veggies and complete the meal with healthy fats or complex carbohydrates.

Take a short twenty-minute break after eating your meal and wait to see if you are still hungry. After twenty minutes, if you still feel hungry then continue to eat more food.

If possible try to eat organic foods as they can be better quality foods compared to non-organic foods.

Simply, organic foods include grass-fed, free range, and hormone free animal products.

If you eat fish like salmon make sure it is "wild, freshwater" salmon and not farmed raised salmon.

Processed sugars should be completely eliminated from the Warrior Diet. In addition, exercise while practicing the Warrior Diet is highly recommended.

Guidelines for Success with the Warrior Diet

Remember to plan your meals ahead of time so that you ensure you eat the right combination of proteins, fats, carbohydrates and vegetables.

Examples of the Good Food Combinations

- Eggs and beans
- Seeds and nuts
- Eggs and sweet potatoes
- Berries and protein
- Sweet potatoes and green vegetables
- Nuts and wine
- Cheese and wine
- Brown Rice and beans

Examples of Wrong Combinations of Food

- Pasta and wine
- Pasta and nuts
- Raisins and nuts (trail mix)
- Sugar and cream
- Jelly and peanut butter
- Jam and bread
- Granola (honey nut)
- Sour cream and potatoes

Warrior Diet Sample Meal Plans: Daytime Options

Remember, the Warrior Diet consists of eating one large meal at night.

However, if you do feel like eating a small snack in the morning or afternoon, below are some healthy options that you can choose from:

Morning or Lunchtime snack:
- Tea (or)

- Sugar free coffee (or)

- one piece of fruit (8 ounces of berries) (or)

- spinach or lettuce salad with tomatoes, peppers, mixed greens, mushroom, onions, sprouts, and cucumber (with small amounts of olive oil)

Warrior Diet Sample Meal Plan: Nighttime Meal

For your one large meal of the day try some of the following food groups:

- **Protein:** Eggs (cooked or poached), wild freshwater fish, organic cheeses such as goat cheese and cottage cheese.

- **Cooked Veggies:** Grilled or steamed cauliflower, broccoli, zucchini, onions, spinach, okra, and mushrooms.

- **Raw Veggies**: Broccoli sprouts, salad greens, as well as red, yellow, and orange vegetables.

- **Carbs:** Sweet potatoes, steel cut oats, legumes, and beans.

- **Fats:** Avocados, olive oil, almonds, walnuts.

Remember to keep in mind that when it comes to eating your one large meal at night, you want to make sure you eat a good variety of proteins, carbs, vegetables and fats.

In addition, you want to make sure you consume enough calories and drinks lots of water so that you can stay full and remain hydrated.

The Warrior Diet is a popular intermittent fasting method because it allows sensible snacks to be eaten during the day.

For the hardcore weight loss junkies, they have the option to skip eating daytime snacks and simply eat one large meal at night.

The benefits that you will get from the Warrior Diet are:

- Tremendous amounts of energy during the daytime especially if you skip the daytime snacks.

- Extreme high levels of alertness as a result of your body using very little to no energy to burn the food that was eaten and digested at night while you sleep.

- You will develop extraordinary discipline with your eating habits as well within yourself.

- You will get good quality deep sleep as a result of eating a very large meal that will immediately tire you and make you want to sleep.

- You will lose tremendous amounts of body fat as a result of fasting for a long period of time.

Every-Other-Day Fasting Method

The every-other-day fasting method was established by an assistant professor, Dr. Krista Varady, from the University of Illinois.

Based on Dr. Varady's research, women should consume between 500 to 600 calories on the days they fast and men should consume between 700 to 900 calories on the days they fast.

However, on non-fasting days, you can eat anything you want and as much as you want.

The following meals can be used on the days you fast:

Chicken Meal
- ½ cup of cooked chicken breast cooked without the skin and topped with lemon juice and fresh-ground pepper
- A bowl of tomato or low-sodium vegetable soup
- 1 ¼ cups of fruit salad

For Men: You can have a large sweet potato with your meal.

For Women: You can have a small sweet potato with your meal.

Lean Beef Meal
- Choose a lean piece of beef like sirloin steak or tenderloin steak.
- Add onions to the steak.
- Spinach salad
- Sweet potato

For Men: Eat 1 large sweet potato with your meal.

For Women: Eat 1 small sweet potato with your meal.

Seafood Meal

It is important to consume omega-3 fatty acids because they are great for your heart and simply good for your overall health.

Here is a short recipe for your seafood meal:
- **For men:** Five ounces of sautéed shrimp with jalapenos, garlic, onions, and some tomatoes (fresh and diced)
- **For women:** Three ounces of sautéed shrimp with jalapenos, garlic, onions, and some tomatoes (fresh and diced)
- 1 cup of brown rice.
- 2 cups of kale or spinach - Flavor the kale/spinach with crushed red pepper, red and garlic.
- ½ of an avocado chopped
- Place it all in a six-inch corn tortilla

The No Meat Meal

For individuals who do not eat meat but still want to practice intermittent fasting they can make a delicious pizza as one of their meals.

Here is what you need:
- Use a whole-wheat pizza crust.

- Use toppings such as black beans, diced tomatoes, barbecue sauce, fresh corn, and shredded mozzarella cheese.

- Have a bowl of butternut squash soup, made using ¾ cup of fruit sorbet and some veggies.

- Add ½ cup of fruit such as blueberries.

For women: reduce your portion size accordingly.

Every-Other-Day Fasting - Meal Planning

Below are some meal recipes that you can use for the every-other-day fasting method.

However, keep this mind, on your low-calorie days or your fasting days women should consume between 500 to 600 calories and men should consume between 700 to 900 calories.

Also keep in mind to modify the recipes to fit your calorie intake.

Now if you exercise on your fasting days you want to increase your calories maybe even double your calories depending on what type of exercise you plan to do.

In addition, you want to make sure you eat healthy complex carbohydrates on the days that you exercise so that you have enough energy to make it through your workout as well to recover from your tough workout.

Every-Other-Day Fasting Recipes

Non-Fasting Days (2 Large Meals)

Recipe 1

Lunch Time
- Make an omelet using egg whites, mushrooms, green peppers, and onions.
- Cook 4-ounce chicken breast
- 1 large sweet potato
- 3 cups of spinach
- 1 cup of blueberries
- Handful of walnuts

Dinner Time
- Sirloin Steak and eggs
- 2 cups of mixed vegetables like broccoli, carrots and peas
- 1 large sweet potato
- 1 whole avocado

Low-Calorie Fasting Day

Recipe 2

Lunch Time
- Small Bowl of steel cut oats
- Scrambled egg whites
- 1 cup of spinach

- Handful of almonds

Dinner Time
- 4-ounce chicken breast

- 1 cup of spinach

- ½ of an avocado

Non-Fasting Days (2 Large Meals)

Recipe 3

Lunch Time
- Hummus with tomato and lettuce

- Whole wheat wraps

- 2 cups of spinach

- 1 cup of blackberries

- Handful of walnuts and almonds mixed

Dinner Time
- Skinless chicken tenders served with low sodium sweet sauce

- 1 large sweet potato

- 1 small avocado

- 2 cups of broccoli

Low-Calorie Fasting Day

Recipe 4

Lunch Time
- Scrambled eggs (include yolk)
- Whole wheat toast
- 2 cups of spinach

Dinner Time
- 4-ounce sirloin steak
- 1 cup of mixed vegetables
- 1 small avocado

Intermittent Fasting Method (5 days of not fasting: 2 days of fasting)

For the intermittent fasting **5 days of not fasting: 2 days of fasting** method you would eat regular meals for five days.

So, for 5 days you will not fast but instead simply eat nutritious meals.

For the remaining two days, you will fast and eat low calorie meals.

For the two days that you fast you can simply fast for 16 hours and have an 8-hour eating window or you can simply do a bit of a Warrior Diet where you only eat one large meal for dinner.

The great thing about intermittent fasting is that it allows you to be flexible with your lifestyle

Keep in mind that for the 5 days that you are eating regular meals, it is important to slightly reduce your carbohydrates.

Only consume moderate amounts of carbohydrates if you plan to do some strenuous exercise.

These are some of the ways of how to manage the **5 days of not fasting: 2 days of fasting** method.

Tips for Intermittent Fasting Method (5 days of not fasting: 2 days of fasting)

- Your hours of eating don't always have to be so rigid.

  Instead, try different eating schedules to see what fits your fasting schedule.

- While fasting you can choose to eat three small meals during your eating window.

  You can also decide to simply have 2 large meals or simply 1 very large meal like the Warrior Diet.

  Remember, the choice is yours to decide how much you want to eat and how often you want to eat.

- When it comes to eating while fasting, you don't have to eat such a wide variety of food.

  Instead narrow down your food choices to a select few healthy proteins, carbs, fats and veggies and focus on eating them day after day.

  Once you get used to eating the same foods every day, you will know exactly how much food you are eating as well as how to control your portion sizes for maximum weight loss.

Maximize the Flavoring of Your Food and Minimize the Calories

- Research shows that eating vegetable soup keeps you feeling full longer than eating a modest serving of vegetables on a plate.

  So, if you decide to make vegetable soup do so by making homemade vegetable soup using natural vegetables.

  In addition, stay away from canned vegetable soup because canned vegetable soup contains a lot of sodium.

- Flavor your foods with spices and herbs such as lemon juice or vinegar for salads.

  You can also use hot sauce to flavor your food.

  Just make sure to look at the food labels and always check the ingredients as well as the calories and sodium listed on the food labels.

- Try to eat more vegetables especially green vegetables.

  Vegetables have very little calories and vegetables like spinach and broccoli contain fiber which will keep you feeling full compared to other foods.

- Eat whole natural foods and stay away from prepackaged foods, canned foods, frozen foods, processed foods and foods in boxes like cereals.

  Simply try to eat as natural as possible. If the food is fresh and natural then eat it!

- When it comes to eating healthy you can grill your food, bake it and you can even fry your food.

  Keep in mind that if you fry your food you should use olive oil or you can simply fry your food without using any oil by using a nonstick cooking pan.

Below is a List of Some Foods for Intermittent Fasting:

- Berries, blackberries or raspberries

- Vegetables like spinach, kale and broccoli

- Baked or Boiled eggs

- Nuts like almonds and walnuts

- Lean meat like chicken breast, sirloin steak or skinless chicken breasts

- Steel cut oats

- Sweet potatoes (powerful source of energy and vitamins)

- Tea or black coffee (no sugar)

The (4 days of not fasting: 3 days of fasting) Intermittent Fasting Method

The **4 days of not fasting: 3 days of fasting** method requires you to fast for three days out of seven days.

So, you will fast for three days and for the other four days you will eat your regular healthy meals without fasting.

Just like the other fasting methods, you should not eat any processed foods, refined foods or foods high in sugar.

If you do eat processed foods or foods with sugar, your body will begin to crave these unhealthy foods so it is best to simply stay away from them.

However, as you condition your body to eat healthier nutritious foods your body will get used to these foods and you will lose your cravings for unhealthy processed foods.

How The (4 days of not fasting: 3 days of fasting) Method Works

As stated before, the **4 days of not fasting: 3 days of fasting** method requires you to fast for three days out of seven days.

The **4 days of not fasting: 3 days of fasting** method does not require you to fast consecutively for three days.

Instead, you can fast every other day or you can fast for one day then the next day can be your non-fasting day followed by two days of fasting.

For example:
- Monday, you will fast.
- Then, Tuesday and Wednesday are non-fasting days.
- Then on Thursday you fast.
- Then Friday is a non-fasting day.
- Then on Saturday you fast.
- Then Sunday is a non-fasting day.

As stated before about other fasting methods, the **4 days of not fasting: 3 days of fasting** method does not have specific days that you must fast for three days.

Instead, the choice is up to you what days you want to fast.

The most important thing is that you fast for three days out of the week.

Here are some results after twelve weeks from a small study group that used the 4:3 fasting method:

- **Fat mass reduction:**   3.5 kilograms with NO loss in muscle mass

- **Body weight reduction:** Over 5 kilograms

- **Reduced blood levels:** 20% reduction of triglycerides. Triglycerides are the main form of fat in the body. So, this means your body fat percentage was reduced by 20%.

- **Leptin levels:**   40% decrease. Leptin is a hormone in the body that is responsible for telling us when we are hungry.

In addition, Leptin is responsible for controlling the body's weight. So, the small study group's hunger as well as bodyweight was reduced by 40% after 12 weeks.

- **Levels CRP:** Reduced levels. CRP is produced by the liver. CRP's levels rise when there is inflammation in the body.

However, after fasting for 12 weeks, it was determined that the small study group's Levels of CRP were reduced.

The (4 days of not fasting: 3 days of fasting) Method
vs.
The (5 days of not fasting: 2 days of fasting) Method

The difference between the **4 days of not fasting: 3 days of fasting** method and the **5 days of not fasting: 2 days of fasting** method is that the **4 days of not fasting: 3 days of fasting** method requires you to fast for three days and the **5 days of not fasting: 2 days of fasting** method requires you to fast for two days.

It is important to state that both fasting methods are great for helping you to achieve your weight loss goals.

In addition, both fasting methods are options that you can choose from when it comes to losing weight with intermittent fasting.

As stated before, intermittent fasting is not a rigid weight loss diet. Instead intermittent fasting is all about losing weight by fasting.

Fasting has so many benefits and there is no one fasting method that is better over another.

However, it is up to you to decide what works best for you.

In addition, you have the option to experiment with different fasting methods.

But, no matter what fasting method you choose to practice the key to success with intermittent fasting is that you remain consistent with your fasting schedule and you make it a lifestyle.

Chapter 8: Tips and Simple Meal Plans

Simple Guidelines to Follow for Intermittent Fasting

Stay in Control: Depending on which method you choose for your intermittent fasting lifestyle, you need to be sure that you consistently follow the fasting schedule.

For example, if you are following the Warrior Diet then you have to make sure you are only eating one large meal a day.

If you are following the Lean Gains Diet, then you simply fast for 16 hours followed by an 8-hour eating window.

Keep Track of Your Calories: Even though you will be eliminating a meal or two while practicing intermittent fasting, you still want to keep track of the number of calories you are consuming every day because if you are not careful, you can easily overeat.

Remember, to lose one pound of fat per week, you have to burn 3500 calories.

Not to lose one pound of fat per week does not mean you have to do a lot of exercise every day.

Instead, you can focus on simply reducing your calories every day while fasting.

In addition, you can practice portion control which means you control the size of your portions or servings.

For example, you can measure your portion sizes using a food scale.

By using a food scale, you will know exactly how much food you are consuming every day.

Stick to Your Chosen Fasting Method: You need to get into the habit of choosing an intermittent fasting method and set a regular schedule for your fasting plan.

Once your body adjusts to the specific fasting method, it will become confused if you try another fasting method.

In the beginning, as you first begin to experiment with different intermittent fasting methods it is ok to change your fasting schedule.

However, once you find a fasting method and schedule that is convenient for you, you want to stick to that fasting method and schedule so that you can get the best weight loss results.

Remember, consistency is essential for a successful fasting plan.

Meals and Snacks
While you are attempting to lose weight on the intermittent fasting plan, you should not feel the need to be hungry no matter which of the fasting methods you decide to use.

Below are some recipes that you can use for your intermittent fasting meals. Some of the meals may not be very filling so you can modify these recipes as you wish.

Lunch

Porridge
- Porridge Oats – You can also use oatmeal or steel cut oats.
- A ½ teaspoon of honey
- Water and Cinnamon instead of milk can be used for the porridge.
- A couple of eggs

- 3 cups of spinach

Tips:
Instead of using milk for your porridge you can use some water to reduce the calorie count. For some additional flavor add just a pinch of cinnamon.

You can also add some healthy nuts to your porridge like walnuts or almonds.

Toast and Beans Small Snack
- 1 or 2 slices of whole wheat bread
- Baked beans – can use black beans or chickpeas
- Lettuce salad
- Handful of almonds or walnuts

Fruity Breakfast Meal
- Blueberries mixed with raspberries
- Steel cut oats
- Almonds or walnuts
- 3 whole eggs

*Mix the berries and nuts with your oats.

Post workout Fasting Snack
- A ½ teaspoon of honey
- 1 small banana
- Handful of nuts (almonds or walnuts)

Apricots and Yogurt Snack
- Chopped apricots

- Greek yogurt (low-fat)

  *Mix the apricots with the Greek yogurt.

Apricots, Greek Fat-Free Yogurt and Mixed Berries Smoothie
- 1 Greek yogurt

- 1 Apricot

- Raspberries

- Strawberries

- Blackberries

*Blend the ingredients as a smoothie for a delicious meal.

Greek Yogurt, Raisons & Almonds Snack
- 1 Greek Yogurt (fat-free)

- A handful of raisons

- Handful of almonds

  *mix the raisons and almonds with the Greek yogurt.

Blueberries, Kiwi, & Greek Yogurt Snack
- 1 kiwi (chopped)

- Blueberries

- 1 Greek yogurt

- Some walnuts

*Mix all the ingredients for a tasty snack.

Raspberry and Cranberry Smoothie
- Add some raspberries

- 7 ounces of cranberry juice

- 1 yogurt

- Add some water if needed

  *Blend and drink

Steak and Eggs for Lunch
- 1 sirloin steak

- 2 large scrambled eggs

- 1 medium size sweet potato

- 1 small avocado

- Small bowl of spinach

Scrambled Eggs and Steak with Mushrooms
- 1 T-bone steak topped with mushrooms

- 2 large scrambled eggs

- 1 medium size sweet potato

- Salad served with vinegar

Spinach Omelet
- 3 cups of spinach

- 3 medium size eggs

- A small bow of blackberries

- 1 or 2 slices of wheat toast

Instructions

1. Simply, beat or whisk the egg and place in a frying pay.

2. When the bottom is cooked, add spinach to the top and grill.

3. If you want, you can add some herbs, salt, or pepper for additional flavoring.

Oatmeal Pancakes

- 1 Cup of oatmeal

- 1 cup of low fat milk

- 1 cup of All-purpose flour

- 3 scrambled eggs

Instructions

Mix the oatmeal, milk and flour together in a large bowl.

After mixing well, pour the batter onto a pan and cook delicious oatmeal pancakes.

Serve the pancakes with scrambled eggs.

Spicy Stir Fry Chicken

- Tenderloins or chicken breast chopped to small pieces

- 2 cups of broccoli

- 1 large sweet potato

  *Add broccoli to stir fry chicken and mix

  **Add low calorie hot sauce to stir fry chicken for flavor

Snacks

Snack time doesn't always have to be boring. You can have your favorite snack using portion control or simply use a small plate.

Here are some snacks that can be used as desserts with your intermittent fasting meals:

- Some dark chocolate with some raspberries

- Some dark chocolate with a handful of walnuts

- Dried figs and blueberries

- Cocoa powder mixed with skim milk for delicious chocolate milk. This is a good post workout drink.

- Low fat chocolate ice-cream with raspberries

- Low fat vanilla ice-cream with blueberries

These are just a few tasty snacks you can include as part of your intermittent fasting diet plan.

Just remember to consume these tasty snacks in moderation and always focus on maintaining good healthy eating habits.

Conclusion

Thank for reading *"Intermittent Fasting: The Smart Way to Losing Weight!"*

I hope this book provided you with the understanding of intermittent fasting.

In addition, I hope you were able to learn different intermittent fasting methods that you can apply to your life.

It is important to state that making a commitment to change the way you eat is extremely important for losing weight.

What is more important and what has been stated over and over again throughout this book is consistency.

To get the best weight loss results with intermittent fasting you have to remain consistent with your fasting schedule.

You simply have to make intermittent fasting a lifestyle.

When you make intermittent fasting a lifestyle, you have more control about the foods you eat as well as when you eat and how often you eat.

If you are convinced that you have what it takes to take full advantage of the benefits that intermittent fasting has to offer, then the next step is to stop reading and to start fasting.

Simply choose an intermittent fasting method that is convenient for you and give it a try.

Try not to become discouraged if you don't receive immediate results. Instead, experiment with different intermittent fasting methods until you find one fasting method that fits your needs.

Above all, don't rush the weight loss process but instead learn from it and see what works best for you and stick to it.

Last, if you like this book, please recommend it to others so that they too can change their lives with intermittent fasting.